Sameh Rzigui
Sana Bekri
Mohamed Ben Yaala

Bruxism: from diagnosis to prosthetic management

Sameh Rzigui
Sana Bekri
Mohamed Ben Yaala

Bruxism: from diagnosis to prosthetic management

Drawing up a treatment algorithm for bruxing patients undergoing prosthetic rehabilitation

ScienciaScripts

Imprint
Any brand names and product names mentioned in this book are subject to trademark, brand or patent protection and are trademarks or registered trademarks of their respective holders. The use of brand names, product names, common names, trade names, product descriptions etc. even without a particular marking in this work is in no way to be construed to mean that such names may be regarded as unrestricted in respect of trademark and brand protection legislation and could thus be used by anyone.

Cover image: www.ingimage.com

This book is a translation from the original published under ISBN 978-620-6-72928-0.

Publisher:
Sciencia Scripts
is a trademark of
Dodo Books Indian Ocean Ltd. and OmniScriptum S.R.L publishing group

120 High Road, East Finchley, London, N2 9ED, United Kingdom
Str. Armeneasca 28/1, office 1, Chisinau MD-2012, Republic of Moldova, Europe
Managing Directors: Ieva Konstantinova, Victoria Ursu
info@omniscriptum.com

Printed at: see last page
ISBN: 978-620-3-52736-0

Bruxism: from diagnosis to treatment
Prosthetic management

Contents

Introduction

Bruxism has been defined by the American Academy of Sleep Medicine as "repetitive jaw muscle activity characterized by clenching or grinding of the teeth and/or tilting or thrusting of the mandible .[1]

It is described as a common phenomenon, with prevalences of 8-31% for generic bruxism, 22-31% for awake bruxism (AB), and 13% for sleep bruxism (SB) in adults. In particular, there is no difference between men and women, and this prevalence decreases with age. High prevalences are also observed in children and adolescents (e.g., 3.5% to 40% for SB) . [47]

The etiology of bruxism is still a matter of debate, with theories on peripheral factors in bruxism controversial in the current literature... Currently, a consensus is emerging that they play only a minor role and that central mechanisms, in particular the basal ganglion network is responsible .[52]

The consequences of bruxism on the dentition often require the practitioner to establish a prosthetic treatment. In addition to restoring function and aesthetics, this prosthetic treatment needs to be reinforced by a cognitive-behavioural approach.

The practitioner therefore needs to understand the mechanisms of this pathology in order to understand its dangers.

Patients will need to be made aware of their para-functional activity, and educated in how to modify their behaviour, as well as in the use of complementary therapies. Finally, monitoring will play a major role in maintaining the occlusal relationships chosen for the prosthesis in place.

In this context, we discuss and detail the prosthetic management of bruxeur patients through a clinical case study.

In the discussion section, we present our treatment options and draw up a treatment algorithm for bruxing patients who are candidates for prosthetic rehabilitation, with reference to the studies presented in the literature.

Clinical observation

1. Anamnesis:

This is a 70-year-old patient in good general health, consulting the removable partial denture service at the Monastir dental clinic for aesthetic and functional reasons.

The patient reports daytime and especially nocturnal grinding of the teeth, indicating the presence of bruxism.

2- Endobuccal examination :

Endobuccal examination reveals :

Maxillary

The teeth present are: 14, 13, 12, 11, 21, 22, 23, and 24.

Wear veneers reaching half of the teeth present with mylolysis and cracks.

All teeth have a CR/ RR ratio of less than 1, are free of any mobility and are endodontically treated with sufficient endodontic therapy.

The palate is moderately deep and broad. The edentulous crest is rounded, moderately high and broad. The tuberosities are well formed and covered with adherent fibro-mucosa.

At the mandible

Missing teeth are 36, 37, 46 and 47. Wear facets are present on all teeth, with mylolysis and cracks. All teeth have a CR/ RR ratio of less than 1, with no mobility.

The edentulous ridge is rounded, moderately high and wide. The eminences are well-formed and covered by adherent fibromucosa. (fig.1)

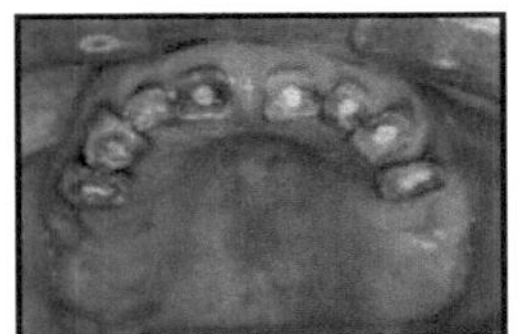

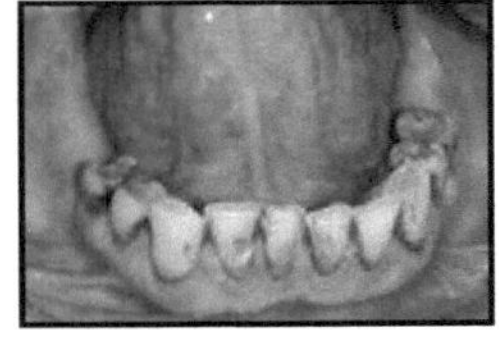

Figure 1:a- Maxillary arch b- Mandibular arch

Examination of the panoramic X-ray reveals a CR/RR<1 ratio for all teeth except 15, 16 and 17, which have already been extracted.

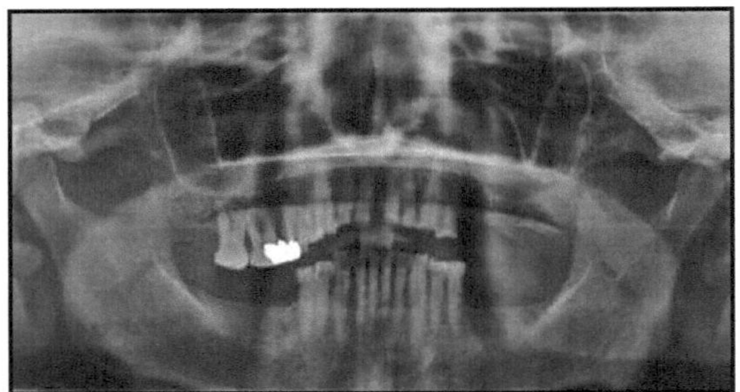

Figure 2: Panoramic radiograph before extraction of irrecoverable teeth

3- Examination of occlusion

DVO is slightly collapsed and PIM is not preserved.

The PO is disrupted by tooth abrasion, the EPD is insufficient and the anterior guide is dysfunctional. (fig. 3)

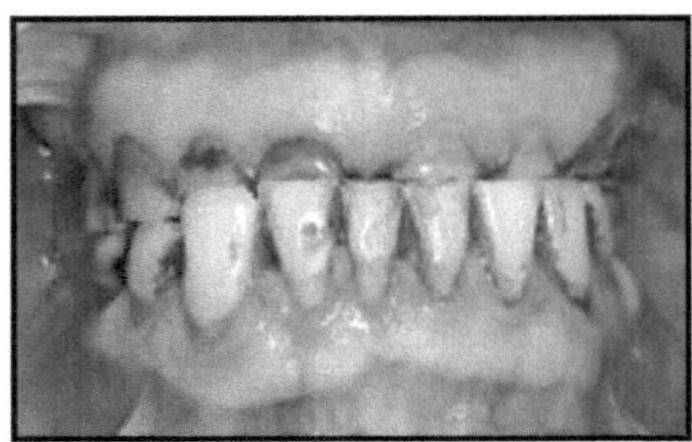

Figure 3: Occluded arches

4- Prosthetic diagnosis

-Patient aged 70, in good general health, consulting the removable partial prosthesis department at the Monastir dental clinic for aesthetic and functional reasons;

-Kennedy Applegate Class I maxillary medium and mandibular low;

-The dentoparodontal and osteomucosal factors are favorable;

-DVO is slightly collapsed and PIM is not preserved.

-The PO is disturbed by tooth abrasion.

-EPD is insufficient. Anterior guide is dysfunctional.

5. Prosthetic decision

Maxillary: Attachment composite prosthesis (twin crowns from 14 to 24 with two extra-coronal Ceka Preci-line® articulated attachments).

Mandible: Simple composite prosthesis (CCM twin crowns on 34,35 and 44,45)

To solve the problem of the reduced vertical prosthetic space available in relation to the fixed prosthesis, the prosthetic project was carried out with a 3mm increase in DVO at the level of the articulator's incisal stem.

This is possible because the patient is normodivergent and the TMJs are healthy.

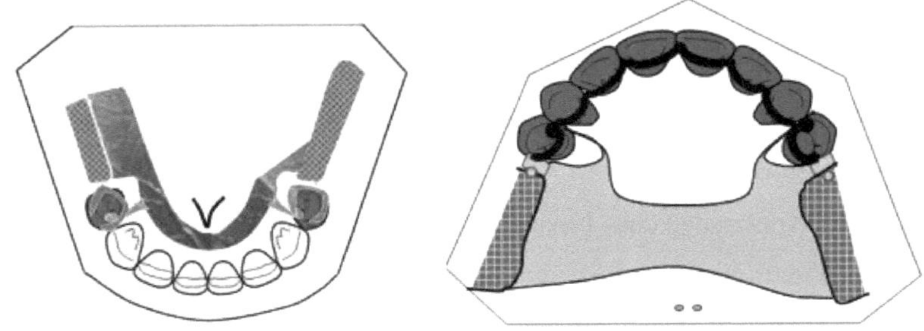

4 a - Mandibular frame design 4 b - Maxillary frame design

Figure 4: Prosthetic design

This decision was embodied in a prospective model (diagnostic wax and master plan). (fig. 5.)

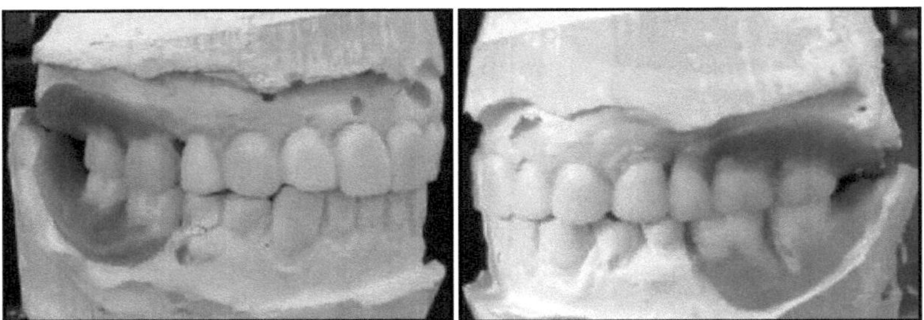

Figure 5: Wax up and guide assembly

6-L he main prosthetic steps:

6-1- Cognitive-behavioral treatment :

The aim of this treatment is to reduce stress on structures (dental, articular, muscular, tendinous) and release muscular tension. The patient must learn to rest the mandible.

This cognitive-behavioural approach is based on the following principles:

Changing a habit is essentially a question of motivation (desire, understanding your problem) and perseverance. You need to gradually replace a harmful habit with a good one. This is achieved by almost constant repetition of the same exercise sequence (reconditioning). It's only during the day, consciously, that unconscious reflexes can be modified.

The sequences of this approach are as follows:

a. **Mandibular resting posture**

Lips touching, teeth not touching, tongue resting lightly on palate (behind incisors). Without pressure on the teeth, breathe through the nose.

b. **Swallowing**

Gently bring all teeth into contact, with the tongue pressed to the roof of the mouth.

Never place your tongue between your teeth or press it against your teeth when swallowing, never tense your lips or clench your teeth.

c. **Release by returning to mandibular resting posture**

-It is essential to use a visual conditioning method: the green reminder dot.

- Each time the eye sees the green dot, this triggers an exercise sequence. In this way, a new conditioned reflex is created, and the patient gradually acquires a spontaneous resting posture, as frequent as possible during the day. This will have a positive effect at night.

A favorable result was obtained after 8 weeks.

6-2 Prosthetic steps :

-Coronal elongation on 11 and 21.

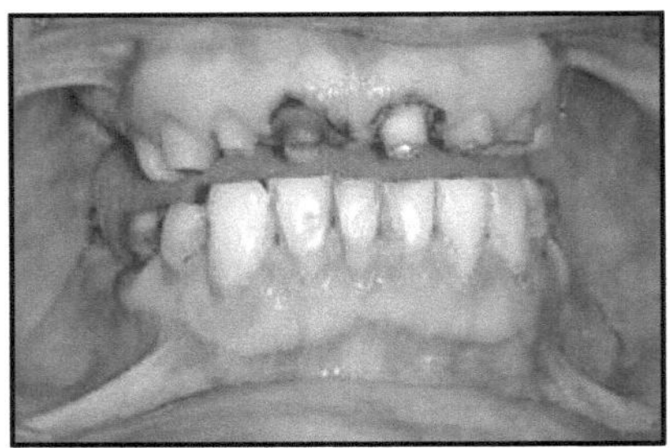

Figure 6: Coronary elongation on 11 and 21

Corono-root reconstructions on maxillary teeth: Fibrous posts and reconstructive resin.

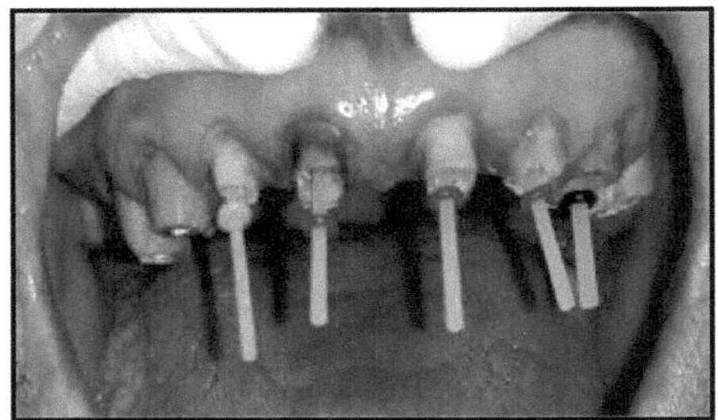

Figure 7: RCR: Fibrous posts and reconstruction resin.

Provisional prostheses are produced by isomolding the wax-up and polymerizing the master framework (fig. 8).

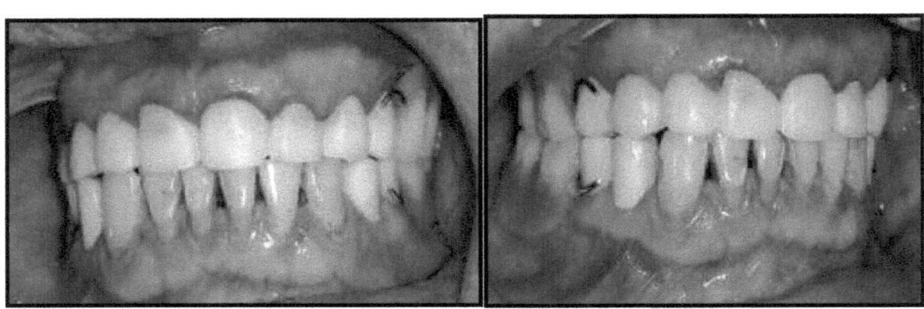

Figure 8: Fixed and removable provisional dentures in the mouth

Global impression taking using commercial impression trays and high- and low-viscosity silicones (fig. 9)

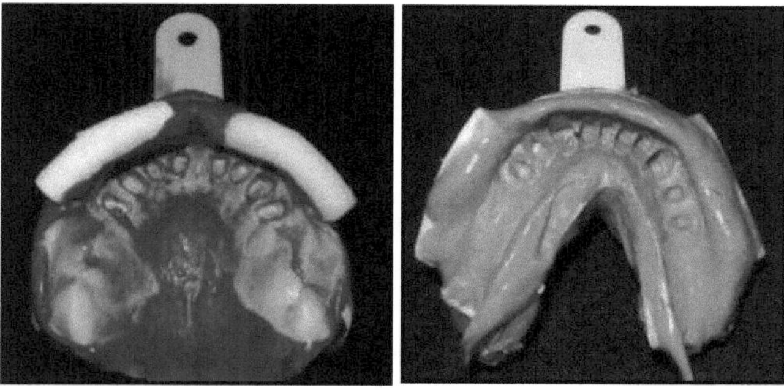

Figure 9: Global footprints

Recording of DVO and centric bite ratios on a semi-adaptable articulator:

We began by determining the anterior occlusal plane, using a bite model covering the prepared teeth and referring to anatomical landmarks: 2mm from the upper lip, and parallel to the bi-pupillary plane. The pronunciation of F's and

In the "V" position, the upper bead should touch the lower lip at the dry-lip/wet-lip junction. The posterior occlusal plane is oriented parallel to Camper's plane.

Once the maxillary cast has been mounted, we proceed to determine the DVO, which in this case has already been predetermined by the master cast. The actual recording was made in centric relation, with both models placed in the mouth at the correct DVO.

Mounting the mandibular cast on an articulator is the final stage of bite registration.

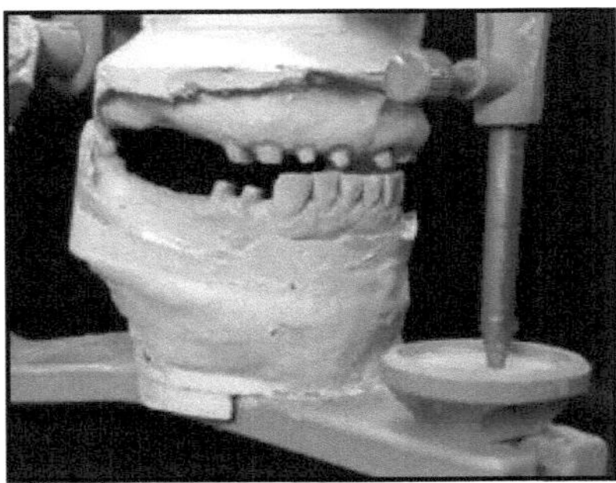

Figure 10: Bite registration

-Design of metal frameworks for fixed prostheses dictated by the design of removable prostheses.

In-mouth fitting of metal frameworks.

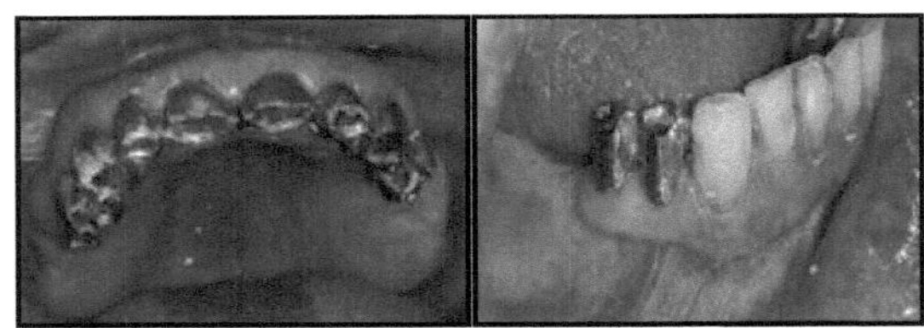

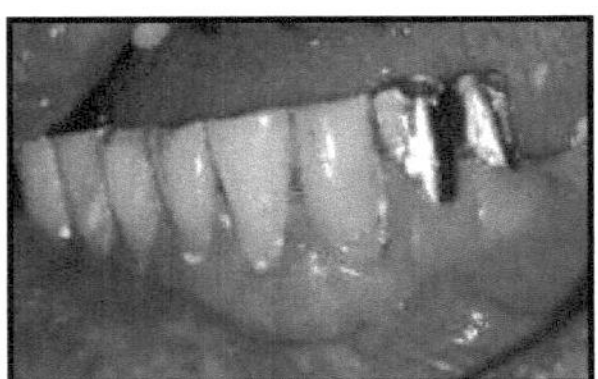

Figure 11: Fitting steel reinforcement

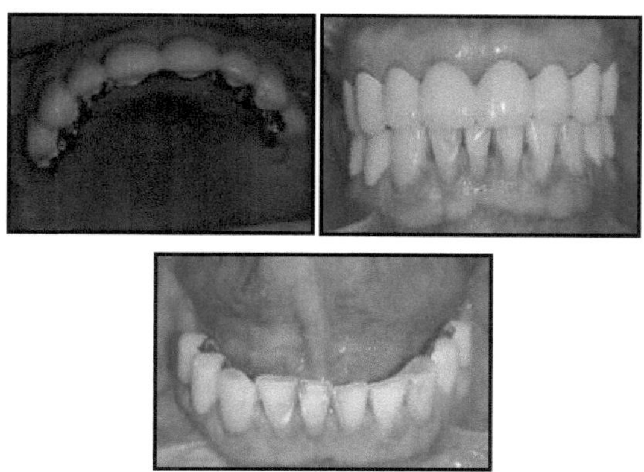

Figure 12: Testing ceramic in the bisque state

-Anatomo-functional impression of the maxillary situation, supported by an individual impression tray and polyether.

- Anatomical mandibular impression using a commercially available impression tray and high- and low-viscosity silicone in simultaneous double-mixing.

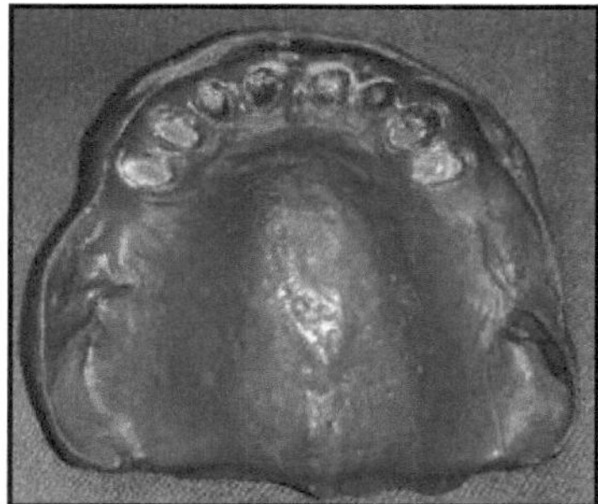

Figure 13: Maxillary situation impression

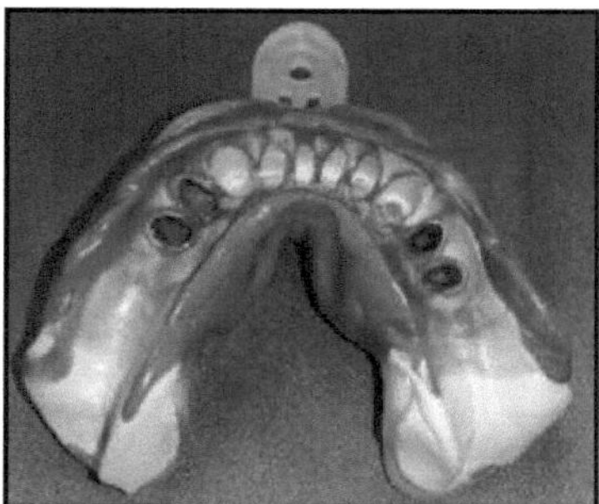

Figure 14: Mandibular situation impression

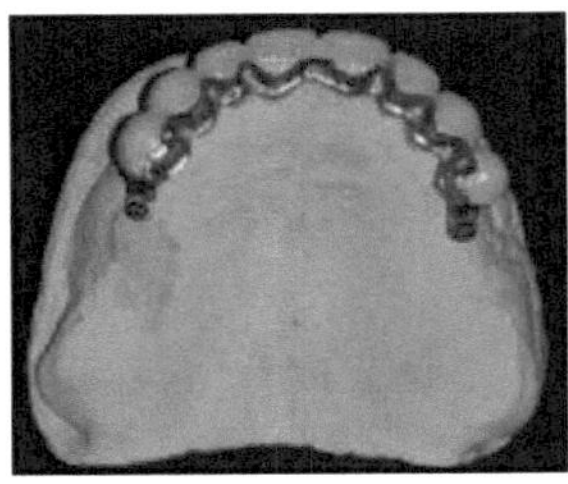

Figure 15: Maxillary working cast

-Frame fitting: insertion, adaptation, stability, retention and occlusion were tested and validated.

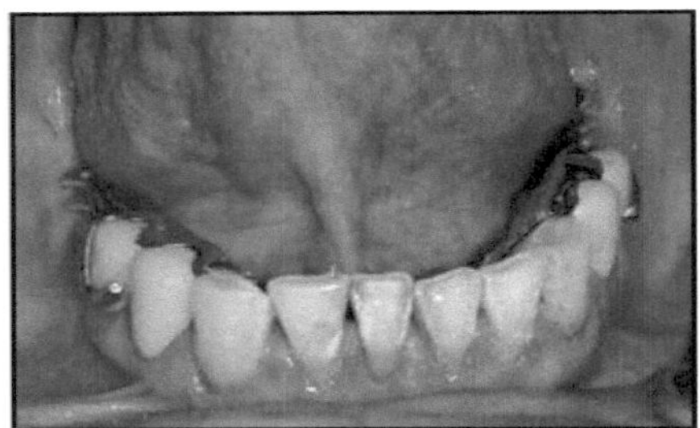

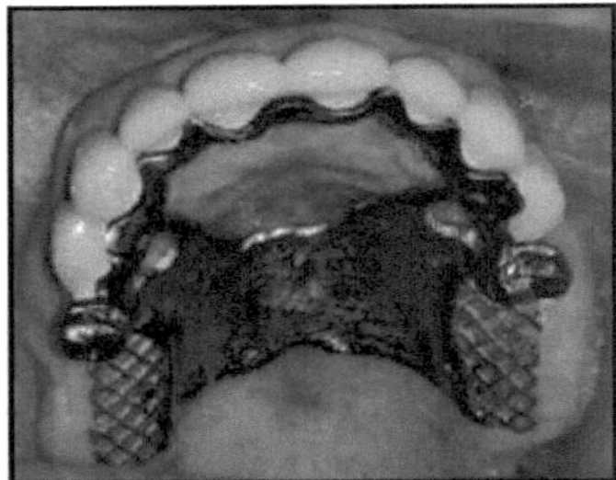

Figure 16: Fitting metal frames

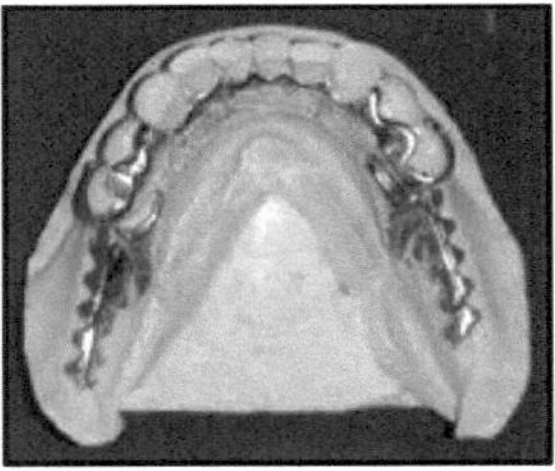

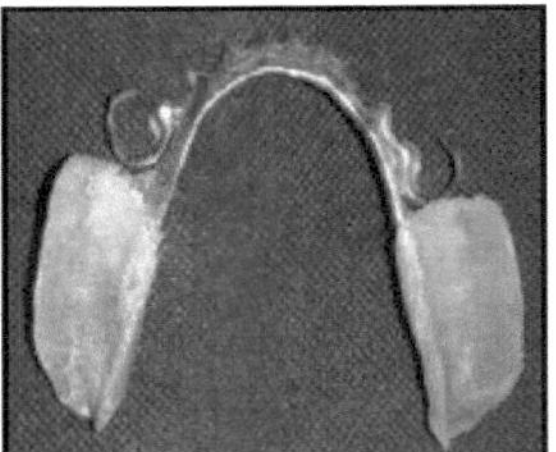

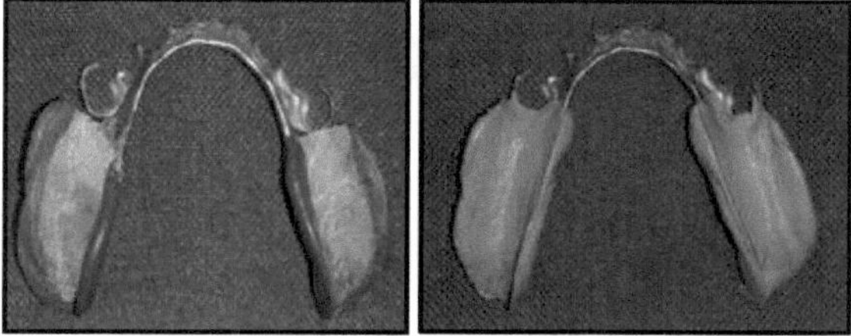

Figure 17: Sectoral anatomical-functional impression stage

-Bite registration and prosthetic tooth color selection

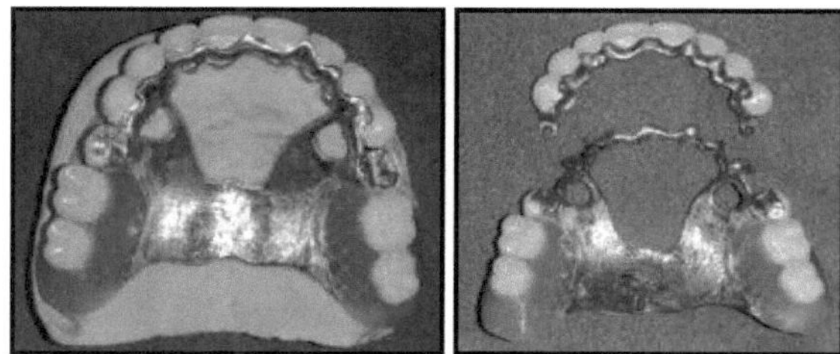

Figure 18: Maxillary composite prosthesis

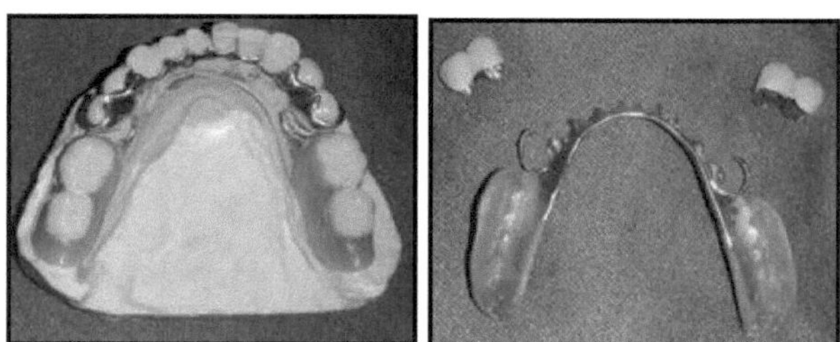

Figure 19: Mandibular composite prosthesis

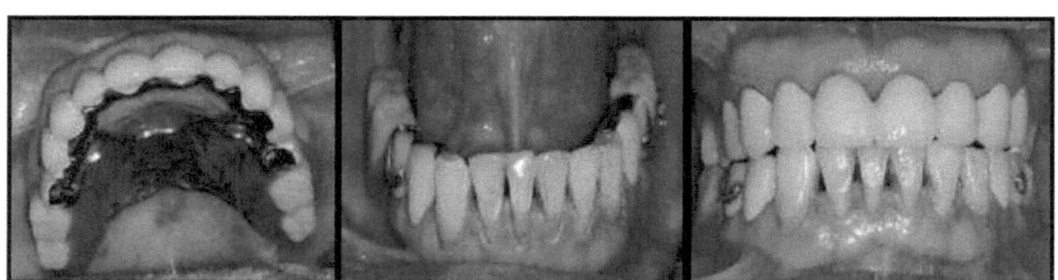

Figure 20: Dentures in the mouth

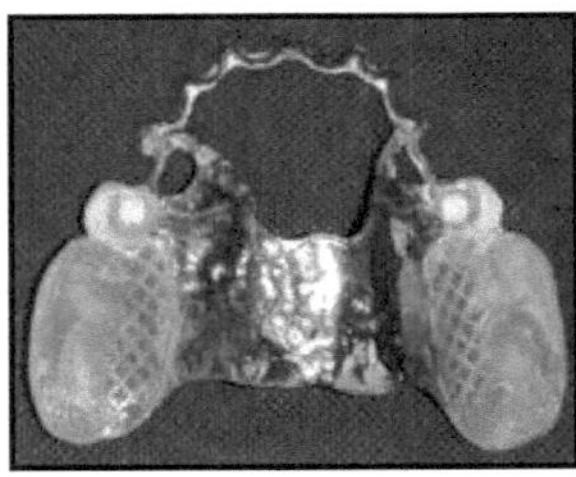

Figure 21: Placement of extracoronal attachments

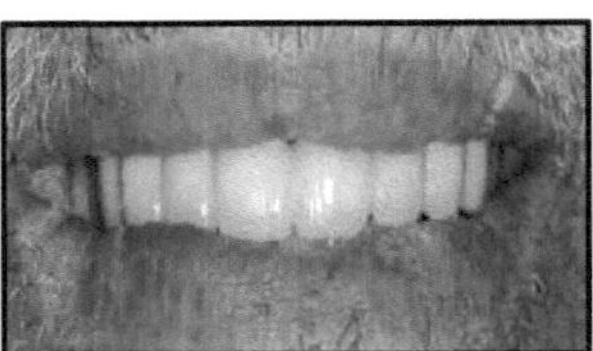

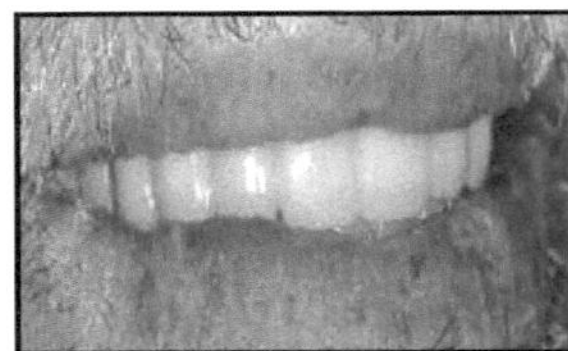

Figure 22: Final result

A splint was applied at the end of treatment to protect the prosthetic reconstructions. Regular follow-up was instituted to support the patient in the management of bruxism and to check the durability of the prosthetic restoration (fig.23).

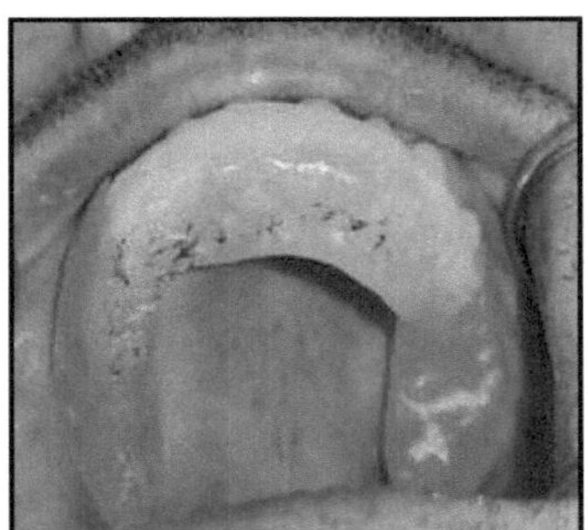

Figure 23: Protective mouth gutter

Discussion

1- How to identify bruxism?

1-1-Diagnostic criteria for bruxism

The diagnosis of bruxism is based on a personal interview with the patient, and will be completed by a series of clinical examinations.

It's essential to distinguish between the different methods of clinical examination. In fact, there are different tests available to establish the diagnosis:

- Self-questionnaire and questioning
- Clinical examination (exo buccal and intraoral)
- Specific devices
- Polysomnography

1-2- Medical questionnaire and patient interview

The individual interview is based on the synthesis of subjective information. By gathering both subjective and objective information, the practitioner can fine-tune his or her diagnosis.

1-2-1- Self-evaluation

To help patients assess their attitudes to parafunctions, they are given a medical questionnaire. This questionnaire is advantageous in that it engages the patient in the search for his or her pathology.

1-2-2- Interviewing the patient: behavioral considerations

Any interview with the patient suspected of suffering from bruxism is based on the search for subjective information such as :

- Clenching/grinding of teeth during the day and/or night,
- Parafunctions (onychophagia, biting tics)

- Headaches
- Oro-facial and muscular pain (masseter, temporalis, neck muscles).

The interview also includes researching and identifying the patient's lifestyle. The latter is itself likely to generate stress factors (work, divorce, death) which need to be highlighted.

In addition, stimulant consumption (alcohol, coffee, tea, energy drinks, drugs) and medical history information (neuroleptic medications) are also strong determinants to be considered in our analysis.

Finally, information on sleep disorders and respiratory (oral ventilation, OSA) and gastric (GERD) disorders will enable us to refine our analysis and diagnosis.

1-3- repercussions of bruxism and clinical signs to look for

The signs and symptoms of bruxism may occur in combination or at different times. They are obviously correlated with the intensity of the forces involved, the frequency of bruxism and how long it has been going on.

According to RUGH[4] , the individual response depends on a number of factors, starting with the modality of the parafunction. Symptom-free bruxism is probably due to a muscular system that is sufficiently resistant to protect both the joints and the muscle itself.

1-3-1- Dental repercussions

1-3-1-1- Dental wear

It is the major sign of bruxism. This attrition-type wear is caused by friction between two dental surfaces .[(70)]

Tooth wear is physiological and occurs with age and diet. Wear facets can be found on all teeth, both anterior and posterior, and on the functional surfaces .[(70)]

Attrition is the appropriate term for the wear of parafunctional origin encountered in bruxism, testifying to the overloads exerted during bruxism. Wear facets located outside functional contact zones, generated by this attrition, are called bruxo-facets, and are smooth, hard and shiny . (40,70)

We can also find tooth surfaces that show marked but long-standing wear, revealing a history of resolved bruxism.

Such pathological wear is first observed on maxillary canines and incisors, as parafunctional activity is generally limited to a lateropulsion movement. When the functional guides have disappeared, the wear affects the premolars and molars and may extend beyond the middle of the dental crown, corresponding to stage 4 of the classification proposed by ROZENCWEIG(74) . (Tab.I)

Table I: Classification of tooth wear according to Rozencweig et al. (1994)

Classification des différents stades de l'usure dentaire	
Stade 1	Usure de l'émail concernant uniquement moins de 3 couples de dents antagonistes
Stade 2	Usure de l'émail et de la dentine en îlots concernant moins de 6 couples de dents antagonistes
Stade 3	Usure de l'émail et de la dentine sans îlots concernant plus de 6 couples de dents antagonistes
Stade 4	Usure atteignant au moins la moitié de la couronne

Stages 3 and 4 involve a severe form of bruxism with a significant psychological dimension. Rozencweig proposes the term "brycosis" for these last two stages (Brocard et al. 2007).

It should be noted that these dental alterations progress slowly. Interdental contact points become increasingly important, leading to occlusal instability and a sometimes significant discrepancy between the ORC and the OIM.

Widespread tooth wear due to bruxism results not only in a loss of vertical dimension, but also often in advancement of the mandible. It should also be noted that if the bruxer has a preferred side, asymmetrical wear and vertical displacement also occur, leading to joint and muscle imbalance, as well as interference with laterality.

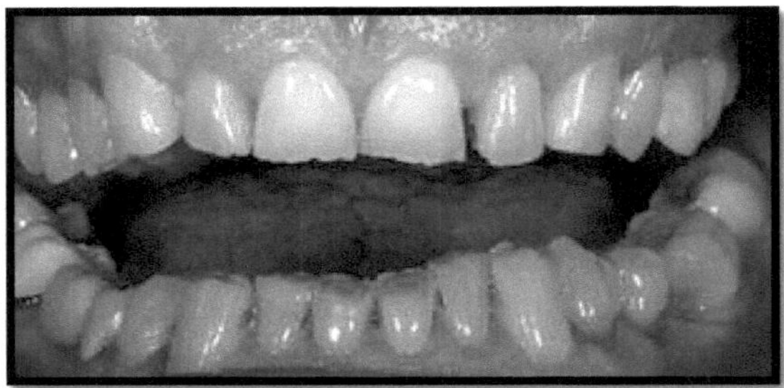

Figure 24: Attrition facet

1-3-1-2- Hypersensitivity

We encounter four degrees of wear when we examine the tooth surface:

- Degree 1: Enamel only ;
- Degree 2: enamel + dentine ;
- Degree 3: dentine ;
- Grade 4: dentin + pulp.

Hypersensitivity is mostly encountered in the last two degrees.

1-3-1-3- Cracks, splits, fractures

Cracked teeth are also a sign of bruxism or bad dental habits. Sometimes difficult to detect, clinical observation must be rigorous. Cracks, fissures and fractures may appear at a more advanced stage.

Clinical findings tend to show that a higher risk can be identified in categories of patients suffering from centric bruxism.

Two-thirds of cracked teeth are mandibular molars. This observation is related to the fact that these teeth, by virtue of their anatomy and location on the arch, are subject to significant occlusal stresses. . [45]

1-3-1-4- Pulp mortifications

Circulatory microtrauma through the apex or microbial infiltration of deep fissures can lead to pulpal mortification. However, this process is chemical and favours concomitant obliteration of the canaliculi, which limits the risk of any septic necrosis or apical periodontitis.

1-3-2- Muscular problems

One of the signs most frequently encountered in bruxing patients is hypertrophy of the mandibular elevator muscles, in particular the masseter muscles. This is why masseter hypertrophy has been adopted by the American Academy of Sleep Medicine (AASM) as one of the diagnostic criteria for subjects suffering from sleep bruxism.

Although it is sometimes used, it is no longer included in the current version of the AASM diagnostic criteria .[(17)]

In fact, this activity is one of the reasons why patients come to the dental practice: they complain of pain, a feeling of muscular fatigue, morning stiffness and sometimes a limitation in opening their mouths when they wake up[(14)] . Muscles subjected to such intense and prolonged contractions become tetanized, leading to an imbalance in cellular oxygenation. Muscle pain is merely the expression of contractures linked to overactivity and fatigue.

It's worth noting that unlike temporomandibular disorders, where muscle sensitivity is often unilateral, myalgias and masseteric hypertrophy, when present, are always bilateral. Even in cases of eccentric bruxism, muscle hyperactivity (EMG) remains bilateral, although it is comparatively higher on one side.

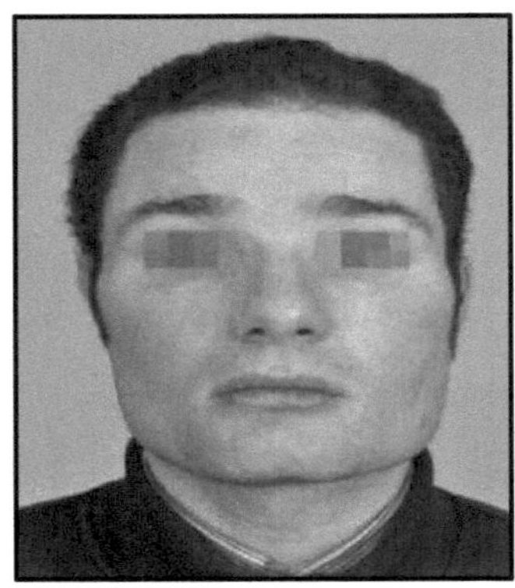

Figure 25: Masseterine hypertrophy developed in bruxism [3]

1-3-3- Joint damage

Although many bruxers suffer from temporomandibular disorders during mastication or even at rest, if left untreated these can worsen, helping to install joint osteoarthritis through mechanical wear of the joint surfaces.

The classic trilogy of mandibular joint disorder (MJD) [73] is presented by BAD:

- B: Articulation sounds, reflecting variations in condylo-disc ratios.
- A: Pain, (correlation with bruxism can be demonstrated by pairing two antagonistic bruxo-facets and holding pressure for a few minutes, usually sufficient to trigger the painful attack).
- D: Dyskinesia.

Although a significant correlation between bruxism and neuromuscular dysfunctions has been observed in adolescents, authors have differing opinions as to the causal link between these and bruxism itself. According to LOBBEZO and LAVIGNE, the relationship between bruxism and temporomandibular disorders is unproven. .[48]

Nevertheless, it should be noted that a joint examination is necessary for every patient suffering from bruxism, in order to take into account any joint disorders in the proposed treatment.

1-3-4- Periodontal problems

❖ **Widening of the desmodontal space :**

This enlargement is simply due to the fact that the viscoelastic capacity of the teeth has been exceeded by intense clenching.

❖ **Dental mobility:**

For some authors (Glaros and Rao, 1977; Pavone et al., 1985), they could be linked to an enlargement of the ligament space, secondary to frequent occlusal trauma in the absence of any periodontal disease; conversely, in the presence of advanced periodontal lesions, tooth mobility in one or more teeth can represent a real painful alarm during occlusal contacts. If, however, this pain is violated during bruxism, the process of tooth loss will be too rapid . (12, 58,89)

❖ **Bone and gum signs :**

In the absence of periodontal disease, and where occlusal forces are well distributed, they will provoke a periosteal reaction, making the alveolar bone appear denser. This can lead to hypercementosis, thickening of the alveolar gingiva (Mac Call's festoons and Stillman's fissures), and pain in the alveolar walls.

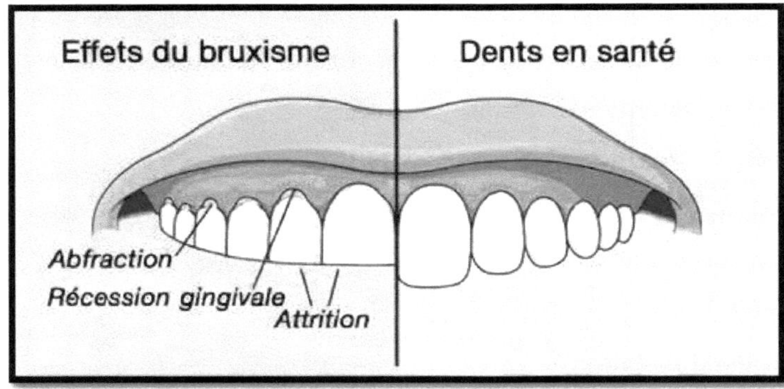

Figure 26: Effects of Bruxism

Exostosis of the gonia angles may also be found, accompanying masseteric hypertrophy. It is visible on the panoramic dental X-ray.

Bone resorptions are possible at the insertion of the medial pterygoid and masseter muscles (Duminil et al 2015).

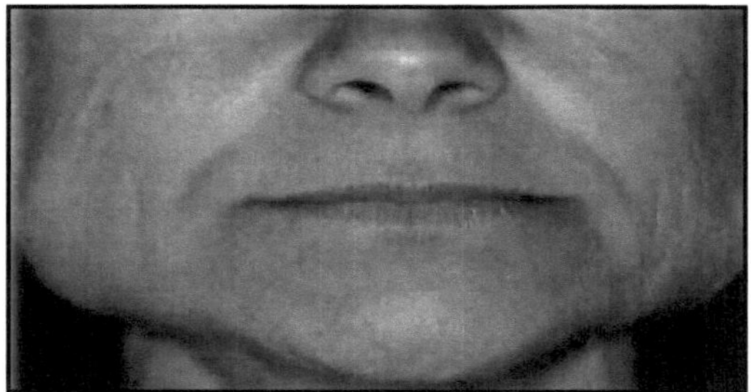

Figure 27: Exostoses of the gonia angles .

1-3-5- Modification of the vertical occlusal dimension

In chronic bruxers, the vertical dimension is often maintained. Tooth wear is often slow, giving the bone time to compensate for the loss of tooth height. The forces imposed will stimulate the bone, increasing bone density. The lower height of the face is therefore maintained[11] , which would complicate prosthetic rehabilitation, necessitating an increase in DVO in most cases.

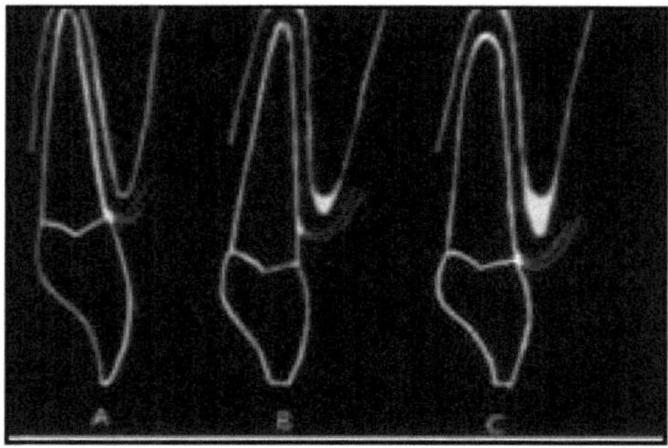

Figure 28: Diagram of bone apposition as a function of tooth wear[8]

However, in some cases, the vertical dimension may not always be maintained, particularly where tooth wear is faster than bone compensation. In such cases, the vertical dimension is lost, resulting in an anterior rotation of the mandible, often accompanied by an end-to-end occlusion and sometimes even an inverted anterior bite, describing a concave profile with an anterior projection of the chin .[16]

1-3-6- Mucosal damage

- **Linea alba:**

The Línea alba, bite line or occlusion line, is characterized by a whitish line of hyperkeratinization. Kampe and D'Incau attribute its presence to bruxism .[17]

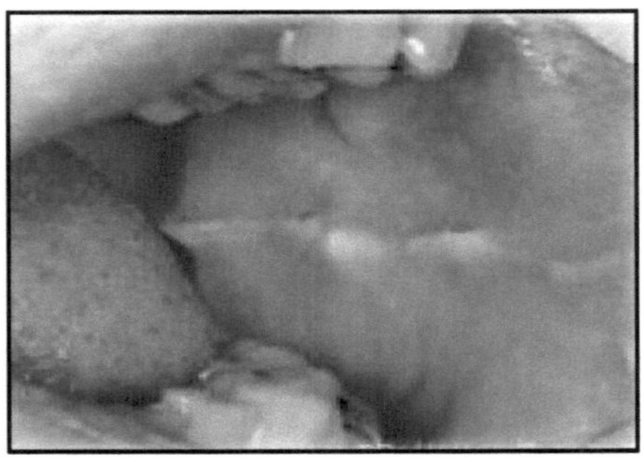

Figure 29: Línea alba described in the context of bruxism

❖ Lingual indentations and bites

Clinical examination of the buccal mucosa in a subject suffering from bruxism may reveal signs of biting, particularly on the inside of the cheek, as well as indentations on the lateral edges of the tongue.

Authors (Sapiro 1992; Kampe et cool 1997, Yanagisawa K et al. 2017) establish a link between the clenching inherent in bruxism and the dental impressions found on the lateral edges of the tongue.

Excessive and regular pressure of the tongue on the palate and teeth can also explain a burning sensation experienced by the patient(fig.).

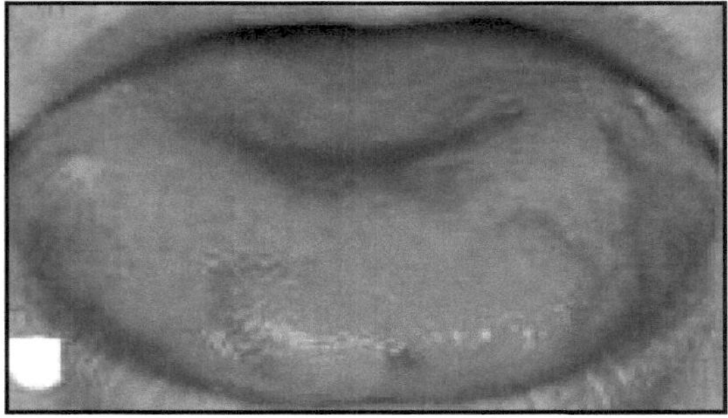

Figure 30: Bites on the tongue in the context of bruxism [33]

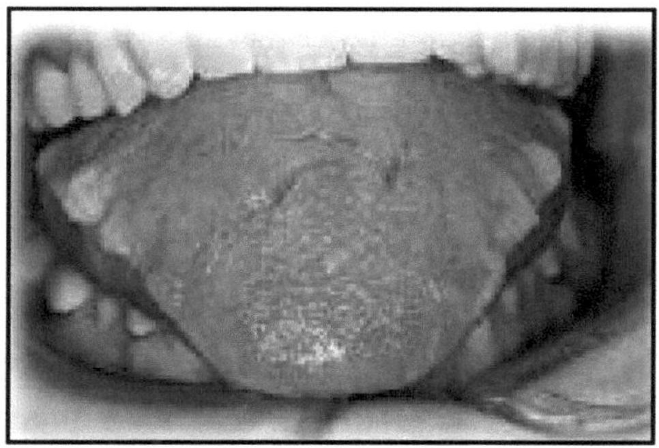

Figure 31: Indentations on the tongue caused by forced compression of the tongue on the lingual surfaces

1-4-Specific diagnostic tools

1-4-1- Intra-Splint Force Detector (ISFD)

The ISFD consists of a splint connected to a piezoelectric film. This wire, sensitive to deformation of occlusal surfaces, provides more reliable results than polysomnography (PSG) [2] .

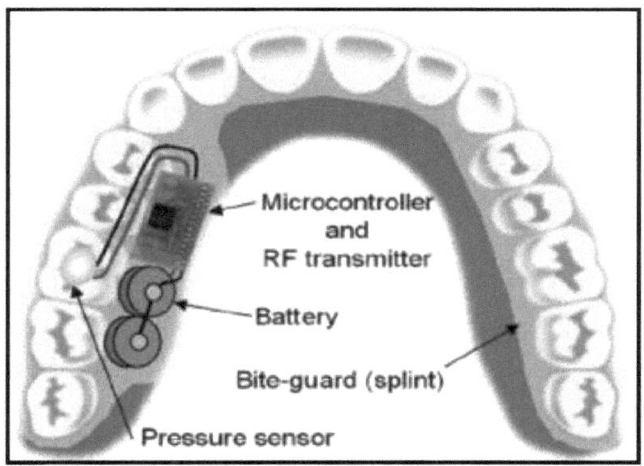

Figure 32: Intra-Splint Force Detector [40]

1-4-2- Brux Checker ® [62,83]

Brux Checker ® is a thermoformable red polyvinyl chloride plate, 0.1 mm thick. Its presentation is attractive due to its low cost and ease of installation. It contributes to the assessment of occlusal stresses associated with bruxism.

Worn for one or two nights, the device can also be worn during the day. Bruxism zones are identified by the supression of red dye.

It is a means of materializing dental behaviors when the patient is unconscious, particularly during sleep. It reinforces speech and motivates the patient to take care of his pathology .[82]

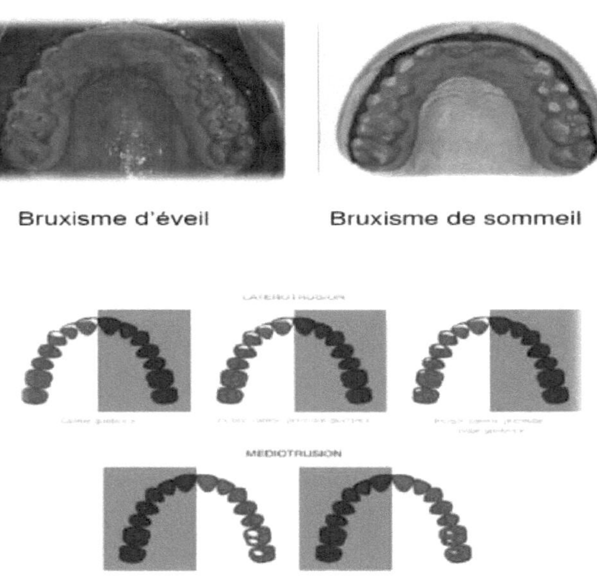

Figure 33: Brux checker

It enables :

- Diagnosis of occlusal patterns based on occlusal contacts during bruxism episodes.
- The patient can visualize his parafunctions and thus make his bruxism a reality.
- Detection of active squeaky patches by disappearance of dye.

1-4-3-Bruxoff ®

The Bruxoff® is a three-channel ambulatory recording device that records EMG activity of the masseters and ECG activity of the heart. It is equipped with three sensors: two placed on the two masseters, and one placed on the chest, held in place by a chest strap .[76]

Recordings are made at night.

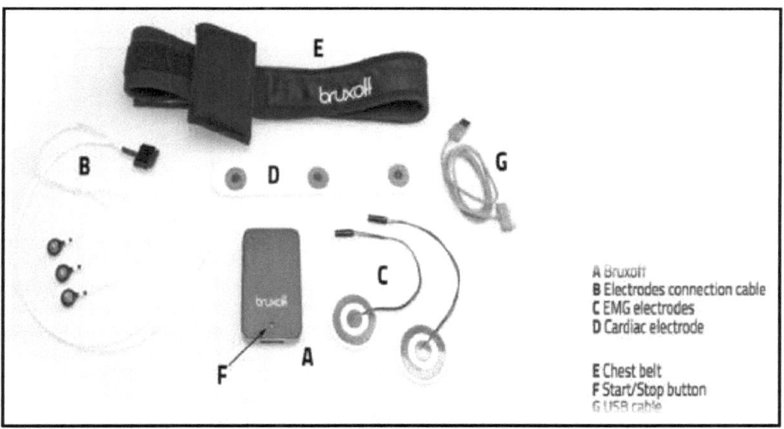

Figure 34: Bruxoff® device

1-4-4- Bitestrip ®

This device is the least expensive (100 euros). It is a single-use device. The EMG electrode is glued directly to the patient's left masseter. The microchip inside the device records the EMG for 5 hours. When the patient wakes up, a number is indicated directly on the device. This value represents the degree of bruxism:

- L: Absence
- (30-60 episodes): light
- (61-100 episodes): moderate
- (> 100 episodes): severe

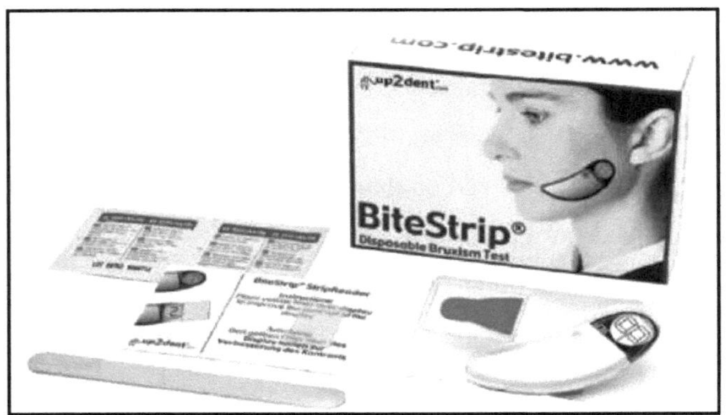

Figure 35: BiteStrip®

1-4-5- Polysomnography [27,39]

Polysomnography is a medical examination in which a patient's sleep is studied within a specific framework. In this examination, the patient's various physiological variables are analyzed: heart rate, respiratory rate, oxygen saturation, brain activity, occulogram. While the patient is asleep, the recording of these different variables is accompanied by a video that enables the patient's behavior to be analyzed.

Polysomnography is thus considered the most reliable and objective diagnostic test for sleep bruxism. It can also be used to determine the degree of severity of the bruxism pathology.

It is also used to diagnose various pathologies, including OSA. On the other hand, this examination is costly and time-consuming. It is carried out in a specialized facility, usually a hospital.

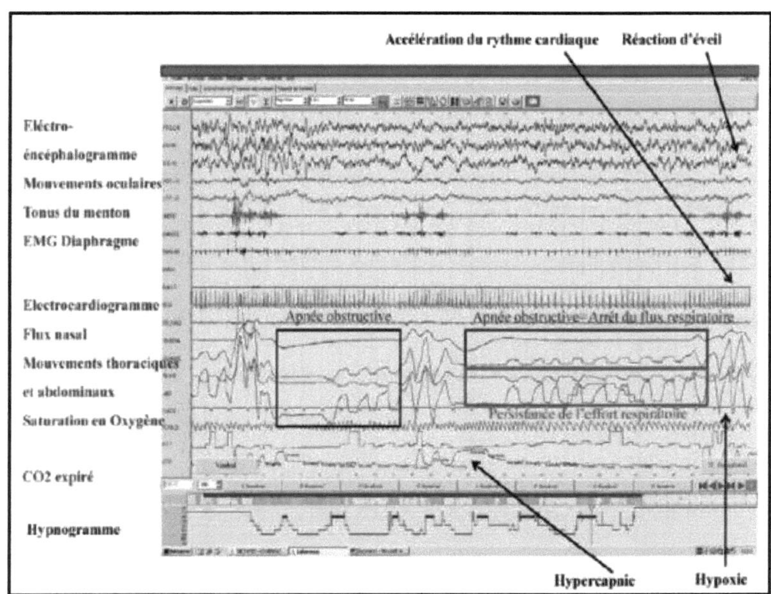

Figure 36: Graphical analysis of polysomnography results.

2-Non-invasive therapeutic approach

As the effect of multifactorial aetiology in the establishment of this pathology is almost self-evident, it is therefore appropriate to begin the treatment or management of bruxism as Rugh calls it[25] with a gentle method involving the patient in the dentist's work:

- Initially, the patient is made aware of his or her pathology and helped to modify the harmful behaviours and habits responsible for the onset or aggravation of bruxism.
- Secondly, the practitioner opts for the indication of muscle reconditioning splints, which remain a simple and effective means of restricting and limiting the effects and consequences of bruxism.
- In the case of an acute phase, the prescription of certain drugs such as benzodiazepines, myoresolvents or antidepressants may be indicated, but this must be done on a limited, well-controlled basis and

sometimes under the supervision of a multidisciplinary team, as the side effects of these drugs are unfortunately multiple.

- The aim of this first phase is to encourage neuro-musculo-articular conditioning, so that prosthetic rehabilitation can be carried out in the best possible conditions.

2-1- Behavioral techniques: self-control of parafunctions

2-1-1 Patient awareness and motivation

It is necessary to convince the patient of the importance of his full involvement in our therapeutic approach and to explain to him that these behavioral habits are deeply rooted in his daily practice, but it is possible to remedy them since the big problem is that they are igonretized by him, so remembering them at every moment helps to get rid of them.

First, the practitioner is asked to explain to the patient the anatomy and physiology of the manducatory apparatus, the modalities of bruxism, its causes and consequences. The patient is asked to make an effort to identify the triggers of bruxism in the course of his or her day and daily life (for example, during stressful moments, in the car or at work).

He should also be alert to feelings of muscle soreness on awakening, signs of bruxism episodes during the night. He will try to distinguish the type of bruxism, i.e. friction, clicking or clenching . (75)

This will make it easier for the patient to be vigilant and fight against his parafunction, reducing the frequency or intensity of inter-dental contact and muscle contracture.

2-1-2-Behavioral rehabilitation of patients

Daytime bruxism is, as previously stated, related to emotional factors. Treatments based on behavior modification are particularly effective in this situation, as the patient's state of consciousness enables him to detect the moment of onset of his parafunction, and the triggers, so he will try to self-limit .[88]

This re-education consists in teaching the patient to adopt a physiological, non-traumatic resting position, in disocclusion with lips together and without muscular tension, as well as relearning physiological swallowing to enable the most appropriate neuromuscular reconditioning possible.

Finally, daily gymnotherapy can be used, with lateral movements to release and relieve musculo-articular tension (8,86).

This is an essential first step, and may be sufficient in some cases.

However, it should be noted that if even after a period of 4 to 8 weeks of this gymnotherapy the results obtained are not significant, this behavioral self-education can be potentiated with treatment by wearing a mouthpiece .[70]

2-1-3-Cognitive approach

2-1-3-1- Biofeedback or Biological Feedback

This is a technique used in medicine, physiotherapy, psychology, etc., which refers to a process whereby an individual learns to modify their physiological activity in order to improve their health and performance . [21, 33,79]

Biofeedback has been reported to reduce bruxism, but the effect does not seem to last after the treatment is stopped. In this method, loud tones are used to wake the patient whenever masticatory EMG activity exceeds a predefined threshold. The patient perceives the awakenings as "punishments" - this is known as "**Classical Conditioning**"[29] .

Another behavioral approach is to include an additional correction each time patients wake up - this is known as "**operant conditioning**". In this case, patients are asked to perform an additional action each time they wake up, such as brushing their teeth. The combination of awakening and correction appears to be more effective than simply waking up .[13]

Other biofeedback methods are currently under investigation, such as the method using a splint system supporting a vibrator that acts on the lip during any bruxism episode .[90]

Very simple techniques are also commonly used to teach patients to monitor their parafunctional behavior and concentrate on not grinding their teeth.

The principle is to establish control reflexes through mnemonic means, such as applying a colored sticker to his watch to remind him to check that he's not tightening, or using stickers, which he affixes to objects visible on a daily basis, such as his cell phone[57] . This creates automatisms and involves him in his treatment plan. He can also relocate and reduce stress by playing with a rubber band, a ball or a ring during each episode.

In this way, the practitioner teaches the patient control techniques to correct their dysfunctions, enabling them to be at the center of their own treatment. This therapy can be an alternative to pharmacological treatment, or an adjunct to psychotherapeutic treatment when it comes to stress management .[33]

2-1-3-2- Transcutaneous Electrical Neural Stimulation (TENS) [4, 72,85]

This cognitive approach is based on the concept of the primordial role of muscle perfusion. Repetition of muscular activity leads to shortening of muscle fibers and, correlatively, to almost permanent contraction. Blood flow decreases, and toxins such as lactic acid accumulate. In this method, patients receive weak, rhythmic electrical pulses transmitted by the nerves that control the muscles of the face. This increases blood flow, helping to eliminate the toxins that cause pain and dysfunction.

Treacy combines TENS with EMG biofeedback to increase mouth opening and decrease muscle tension .[21]

2-1-4- Hypno therapy suggestive

The cognitive approach, during which the patient learns to relax the masticatory muscles, has the effect of reducing EMG activity during sleep. Recent studies confirm that relaxation and meditation techniques have a positive effect on reducing bruxism. The MART [54,68] (Muscle Awareness Relaxation Training) technique enables patients to become aware of their stress through their body's signals. It focuses on posture, muscular contraction and breathing, which, according to studies, leads to a reduction in bruxism thanks to a relaxation of the masticatory muscles, allowing the mouth to open wider, and a reduction in breathing frequency .[88]

One study with 24 participants reported greater efficacy of MART compared to TENS in the treatment of bruxism, suggesting the relevance of relaxation through muscle awareness whole-body and mind training (.[54]

2-1-5- Bruxism and healthy living

2-1-5-1- Power supply

Rethinking your diet can help prevent teeth grinding. Eating carbohydrate-rich industrial products can cause stress, so it's important to adopt a healthy diet. To reduce the risk of jaw cramps, choose foods rich in calcium. This nutrient is known for its calming properties.

Also choose foods that provide a good supply of magnesium. A deficiency in this nutrient makes the body more sensitive to anxiety, fatigue and stress. Stimulants such as alcohol, tea and coffee should be avoided three hours before bedtime. Smoking after 7 p.m. is also strongly discouraged.

2-1-5-2- Physical exercise

Certain sports are recommended to prevent or reduce the symptoms of bruxism.

Relaxing physical activities such as Qi Gong, yoga, jogging, swimming or tai chi reduce the symptoms of teeth grinding.
These exercises reduce muscular tension and improve the state of mind, helping to relieve stress.
Daytime exercise is recommended to reduce bruxism
Effectively. However, intense physical exercise is not recommended after 6 p.m., so that you can return to a calm state at bedtime .[46]
The patient's control of habits, while trying to avoid these destructive practices, is the primary treatment for his or her parafunctions. Some authors advocate the use of biofeedback to treat behavior and habits, before any other treatment. Progress in terms of muscular or dental pain is recorded by the practitioner and regularly reminded to the patient.
It should be noted, however, that these cognitive-behavioural therapies aimed at eliminating certain maladaptive behaviours require a major investment on the part of the practitioner (time, control, follow-up...).

2-2-Pharmacological approach

2-2-1- Regular injections of botulinum toxin (BTX) [56,84]

Botulinum toxin: This is a purified neurotoxin produced by an anaerobic bacterium called "clostridium botulinum", which blocks nerve conduction .[56]

When injected intramuscularly, the toxin blocks the release of acetylcholine at the pre-synaptic level of the neuromuscular junction, causing chemical denervation (ephemeral due to axonal regrowth) limited to the injected muscles. The result is hypotrophy and reduced power and volume of the injected muscle, but no masticatory asthenia with the doses used. [14]
In a study carried out by L. Chikhani and J. Dichamp in 2013 they were able to observe, that:

- Pain subsided completely in 64% of patients after a single injection session, and regressed significantly in 31%.

- Results on mandibular kinematics were satisfactory, with an improvement in the quality and quantity of mouth opening (+8 on average) and symmetrization of mandibular condyle kinetics.
- The results on masseteric hypertrophy are very convincing, with 90% of patients spontaneously reporting a cosmetic improvement in their facial contours, with a reduction in the transverse diameter of the face.
- Results concerning bruxism were positive, with 53% of patients reporting that they had stopped grinding their teeth, and a significant reduction in bruxism without complete cessation in 22% of patients.
- Masticatory comfort was improved in 73% of patients, and a significant increase in the longevity of fixed or removable dental prostheses (crowns, bridges or implant-supported prostheses) was observed in these patients, who rapidly and iteratively deteriorated all prostheses prior to any botulinum toxin injection .(14)

Botulinum toxin injections into the masseter and/or temporal muscles appear to be a highly effective and long-lasting treatment for bruxism, masseter and temporal hypertrophy, and certain forms of algodysfunctional syndromes of the temporomandibular joints .(50)

This treatment, which may seem costly, is certainly less so than so-called "conventional" treatments, since one vial of toxin can treat around two to three patients. What's more, it has no notable or lasting side effects, and can be carried out on an outpatient basis.

The main disadvantage of this treatment is that its therapeutic indication is off-label, as current knowledge of BTX in the treatment of bruxism is based on two RCTs (Randomized Controlled Trials) and a few case reports, so further high-level studies on the effect of BTX on bruxism are needed to establish evidence-based practice of BTX on this issue .(30,84)

2-2-2- Other medicinal substances

A number of studies have looked at the use of drugs to treat bruxism, including benzodiazepines, myoresolvents, SSRI-type antidepressants and anticonvulsants.

Unfortunately, these pharmacological approaches are still under study, and none of them can be recommended for the definitive management of SB.

For example, several studies have shown that the use of antidepressants, including those with sedative properties, can impair sleep by inducing sleep disorders or worsening existing ones.

Regarding our subject Bruxism a study has shown that Venlafaxine: a psychotropic drug used for the treatment of depression, is known to induce or exacerbate sleep bruxism and disrupt muscle tone regulation during REM Sleep . [(92)]

There are very few studies justifying the value of treating bruxism pharmacologically, and the only existing evidence-based data are insufficient to draw definitive conclusions[(93)] . This means that their use can only be very occasional, in the acute phase, and should in any case be limited to a few days to rule out any risk of dependence.

There is insufficient evidence to draw definitive conclusions regarding the effects of various drugs on bruxism. Although some substances related to the dopaminergic, serotonergic and adrenergic systems suppress or exacerbate bruxism activity in humans and animals, the literature remains controversial and based mainly on anecdotal case reports. More controlled, evidence-based research is needed on this under-explored issue.

2-3-Gouttière for muscle relaxation

2-3-1- Definition

It is a device that covers one of the two dental arches, preventing the patient from regaining a habitual maximum intercuspidation occlusion. The splint is an orthopedic appliance, designed to return the patient to a functional orthopedic position, thus restoring all the parameters of physiological position and function. This is one of the key conditions for successful treatment.

2-3-2-Indication of MRM

An occlusal splint can be used to test a therapeutic position[(23)] , prior to any major change for prosthetic reasons, such as altering the vertical dimension[(95)] or creating a mandibular anteposition.

But it is more often used directly as a therapeutic means

An occlusal splint is mainly used for therapeutic purposes .[31]

For some authors (Greene and Laskin, 1972; Rozencweig 1994; Turp et al., 2004), the occlusal splint, by materializing the treatment, would reinforce the "taking charge" effect and act above all as a placebo. However, Ekberg (Ekberg et al., 2003), in a randomized, controlled clinical trial involving 60 patients in 2003, showed that the smooth occlusal splint also acts to resolve contractures .[(24)]

So, while the occlusal splint should no longer be used as a general treatment for DAM, there are still real indications for prescribing it.

2-3-3- Performing the GRM

The gutter should be made of a "hard" material (acrylic resin, to maximize its inhibiting effect). It should be smooth, non-indented and aesthetically pleasing (transparent). [(49,63, 66,71)]

To avoid tooth displacement (egression of antagonist teeth), it is recommended to use a GRM covering the entire supporting arch[(69)] . Contact points should be distributed harmoniously and with the same intensity over the entire arch in centric relationship . [(63,66)]

The anterior guide is functional as a canine guard because this pattern prevents contraction of the elevator muscles on the unworked side . [(69)]

It is advisable to perform MRM in a horseshoe shape to minimize disruption of tongue movements and optimize lingual resting and swallowing posture. In the maxilla, the palate should always be kept clear, with as little encroachment as possible on the retro-incisal support area .[69]

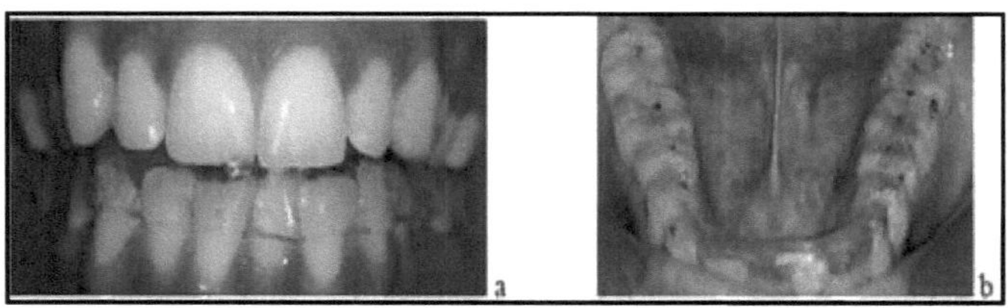

Figure 37: Balanced muscle reconditioning gutter: well-distributed contacts

2-3-4- Choice of support arch :

Should the occlusal splint be made for the maxilla or mandible?

It is probably possible to achieve the same results whatever the occlusal splint situation, but the choice of individual occlusal splint situation depends on a few basic principles. For example, it is essential to always focus on the largest edentulous arch, in order to increase the stabilizing effect by creating additional occlusal contact points. If the incisors are heavily overjeted, as in the case of several Angle II classes, it is preferable to create an occlusal splint on the maxillary arch. In this case, it is difficult to achieve anterior contacts and appropriate guidance with a mandibular splint. Apart from the fact that the mandibular occlusal splint is preferred, it offers the advantage of providing a better resting place for the tongue (which should be physiologically located at rest in the palate). Moreover, in the event of lingual dysfunction, mandibular occlusal splints alter the tongue, which becomes a valuable aid to the practitioner, driving the tongue out of position, forcing it to take up a better upper position[71] . (fig. 38)

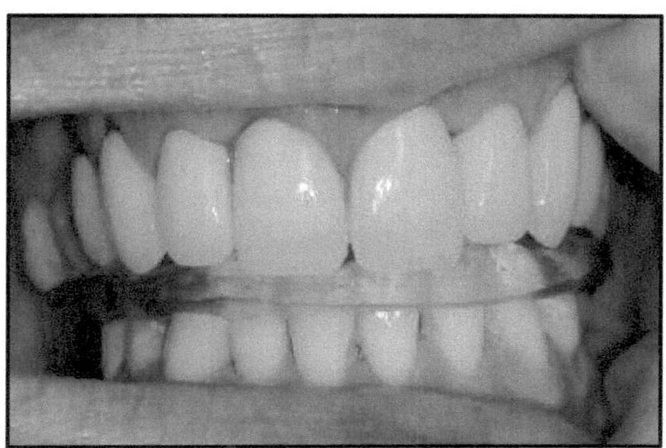

Figure 38: mouthpiece insertion

Table II: Summary of MRM prescription in different clinical situations.

	ARCADE MAXILLAIRE	ARCADE MANDIBULAIRE
INDICATIONS	-Edentement mandibulaire < édentement maxillaire -Classe II/1 d'Angle -Classe I/1 marquée -Contention maxillaire -Bruxeur exagéré -Courbure de compensation accentuée	-Edentement mandibulaire > édentement maxillaire -Classe dentaire I d'Angle -Classe dentaire II/2 d'Angle -Classe dentaire III d'Angle -Ventilation orale -Sensibilité sociale (esthétique et phonation).
+	- Permet la réalisation d'un meilleur plan d'affrontement lisse, d'un meilleur guide antérieur.	-Esthétique -Meilleur confort (diminution de la gêne au niveau de la langue, de la gêne esthétique et phonétique). -Favorise l'ascension de la langue en position haute, contre le palais (avantageux chez les ventilateurs oraux et les patients atteints de SAHOS). -Conservation de la proprioception des incisives maxillaires qui sont chargées de réguler les pressions et les postures mandibulaires. -Libère la suture inter-palatines de toutes contraintes.
—	**Contre-indiquée** chez les patients souffrant de troubles respiratoires du sommeil, tels que le SAHOS.	**Aucune** contre-indication et aucun inconvénient comparé à la GRM maxillaire.

3-Prosthetic treatments

It is essential to ensure that any prosthesis is integrated into and participates in the manducatory functions in the least harmful way possible.

In the case of a bruxing patient, the loss of occlusal landmarks, mandibular posture and reference position, and possibly the presence of functional anomalies in the manducatory apparatus, as well as the major risk presented by excessive forces, can lead to premature destruction of the prosthesis, making diagnosis and prosthetic management of the patient more difficult and delicate.

In order to meet the patient's needs and treatment objectives, and to minimize the risk of failure, it is essential to define a treatment strategy that will enable us to accurately define the most appropriate prosthetic choice. All our treatments (occlusal prosthetic concepts) envisaged to reconstruct the occlusion must be in line with physiology and restore efficient, non-harmful function. Today, the emphasis is on a well-established clinical examination, accurate occlusal diagnosis and morphology adapted to the individual. Emphasizing and diagramming these pre-prosthetic phases will undoubtedly help us achieve our treatment goals . [60,78]

Only an in-depth study can lead to a prosthetic project that meets the following necessary criteria:

- Establish a stable maxillo-mandibular position, using my articular reference, the centric relationship.
- Restore occlusal function by creating occlusal morphologies capable of centering, wedging and guiding.
- Correct assessment of the vertical dimension (has wear altered it to such an extent that it needs to be changed?)
- Ensuring the patient's aesthetic satisfaction, which may be the reason for the consultation [22].

Nevertheless, the practitioner must remember that a prosthesis does not cure the patient of his or her parafunction, and that regular maintenance is essential. Restoring worn teeth without addressing bruxism can only lead to therapeutic failure .[19,61]

3-1- Reminders about occlusion

3-1-1- Reference position, therapeutic position [6, 27,35, 41, 67,94]

The choice of a reference position is a prerequisite for the therapeutic proposal and the subsequent steps. This decision must be taken before the start of any treatment, not during it.

In the case of small endentures, it must be decided whether the patient's maximum intercuspid occlusal position can be used as the design position, i.e. the reference position. In order to give a positive answer, the pre-prosthetic occlusal analysis must determine that this position is stable. A pre-prosthetic preparation aimed at eliminating possible interferences can be considered in order to make this position stable, reproducible and usable as a reference position during prosthetic reconstruction .[7]

3- 1-2- Therapeutic IMO

This is the therapeutic concept that represents the artificial construction model (therapeutic IOM), the result of prosthetic or orthodontic treatment. It aims to restore optimal occlusal functions (centering and wedging) adapted to the patient's particular dento-skeletal structures. Correct therapeutic IOM can be used as a reference position for further treatment.

3-2-Positions with joint reference

The reference articular relationship (RAR), better known as the centric relationship (CR), is defined by a reference condylar situation corresponding to a high, simultaneous, bilateral condylo-disco-temporal coaptation, obtained by a non-forceful control, reiterative in a given time and for a given body posture and recordable from a mandibular rotation movement. It is the reproduction of this limiting physiological joint relationship that makes it clinically interesting. Its existence depends on the pathophysiological state of the temporomandibular joint and masticatory muscles.

Only TMJs and muscles in physiologically functional condition can meet the above requirements.

This reference joint relationship may be natural or stabilized.

- **Natural RC:** the anatomical relationships and physiology of the temporomandibular joints and masticatory muscles are functional and do not result from therapeutic correction or spontaneous healing of a pathological process. The natural RC may have undergone slight physiological adaptation due to age, functional and parafunctional play.
- **RC stabilized** a pathological process has developed in the joint in the past, metaplastic phenomena have enabled functional adaptation resulting in stabilized joint structures. This asymptomatic joint allows reproducible terminal axial movement. The stabilized physiological joint relationship may be the result of treatment of an episode or spontaneous consolidation.

3-3- Criteria for choosing the reference position

Our diagnostic and therapeutic concept is therefore based on the concept of the centric relationship (CR), the starting point for all reconstructive therapies. However, we must bear in mind that this position does not always exist (in the case of a pathological component of muscular, osteo-articular or mixed origin).

In this case, the practitioner is asked to assess the initial clinical situation and ensure that it conforms to a therapeutic classification.

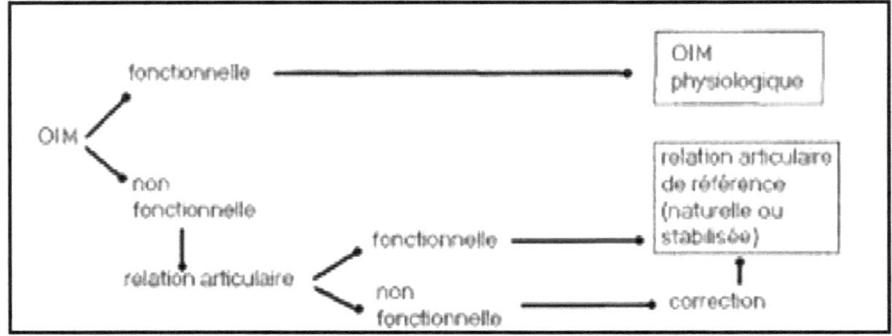

Figure 39: Choice of reference position according to initial clinical situation.

The following questions should be asked by any clinician:

- Is maximal intercuspidial occlusion (MIO) physiological?
- Is the centered relationship (CR) physiological?

When choosing between OIM and RC, a basic rule is applied:

If the IMO can be used as a reference position, the prosthetic reconstruction must be integrated into the existing occlusal scheme. Otherwise, RC is the only option.

The problem is to determine when the IMO can no longer be used as a reference: the pathogenic IMO is considered to be either misaligned or out of alignment.

- **misalignment**: the existing IMO does not match the articular relationship, e.g. contact with an erupted posterior tooth leading to proglation.
- **malpositioning**: the number or condition of the remaining teeth no longer allows stable, reproducible positioning of the mandible.

If the articular relationship is to be used as a reference, it must meet the definition of a functional articular relationship (natural or stabilized). If this is not the case, prior treatment is required to achieve a stabilized articular relationship: this is known as a therapeutic mandibular position.

3-4- Therapeutic mandibular position

In contrast to the reference position, the therapeutic mandibular position corresponds to the desired position of the mandible during treatment. It is not necessarily reproducible, but must be defined in relation to a reference position (e.g.: bilateral propulsion of 1 or 2 mm in relation to the centric relationship: this is referred to as mandibular anteposition).

This position is dictated by the dental relationships already restored in accordance with the chosen mandibular (and therefore articular) position.

Fortunately, however, the reference position and the chosen therapeutic position are often identical. A therapeutic position that differs from the reference position can only be envisaged in cases where the articular relationship serves as a reference; the differential that exists between these two positions can then be appreciated in both directions of the horizontal plane (in the transverse direction: correction of latero-deviation, for example, or in the antero-posterior direction: propulsion, for example).

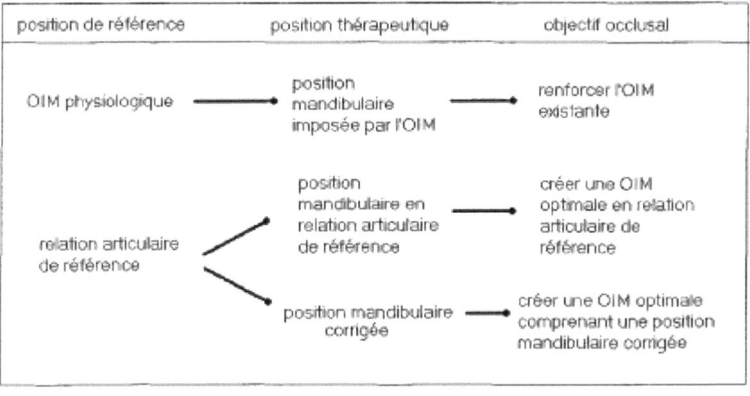

Figure 40: Relationship between reference and therapeutic positions.

3-5- Summary

In summary, the practitioner is faced with four clinical situations:

3-5-1- Functional RC and physiological IMO

The reference position of choice is the IMO; the occlusal objective being to reinforce the existing IMO. However, in the case of complex restorations, this reference disappears, and the use of the reference articular relationship is essential.

3-5-2- Functional RC and pathological IMO

The reference articular relationship is the only usable reference position; the occlusal objective is to create an optimal IOM in the reference articular relationship.

3-5-3- RC disrupted by muscular dysfunction without joint damage

IOM must be corrected by certain treatments (etiological, physiotherapy, pharmacotherapy, behavioral advice, muscle reconditioning splints). The reference position is the RC if the IOM remains non-functional. The occlusal objective is to create optimal IOM in the reference joint relationship.

3-5-4-RC pathology related to WILD (grades 1 and 2)

The therapeutic objective is not disc recapture, but the cessation of painful symptoms by promoting the formation of fibrous healing tissue between the condyle and the mandibular fossa (neo-disc). The occlusal objective is to create an optimal IMO, imposing a corrected mandibular position (PMC). The new "therapeutic" joint relationship is then the reference position.

The reference position corresponds to a condylar position belonging to the reference plane, constituting the zero point of the orthonormal reference system. It must be reproducible, and is referred to as Maximum Intercuspid Occlusion (MIO) or Centric Relation (CR).

The therapeutic position is the desired condylar position of the mandible, while reinforcing the existing IMO, or creating a new one.
Reference and therapeutic positions are confused, unless a corrected mandibular position (PMC) or therapeutic mandibular position (PMT) is chosen.

3-6-Vertical dimension of occlusion (VDO)

3-6-1- Definition(DVO)

The vertical dimension of occlusion corresponds to the height of the lower level of the face when the teeth are in maximum intercuspid bite (MIO).
For the DVO to be estimable, the natural teeth must be able to come into contact with each other, and must be able to ensure the stability of the occlusion and therefore of the mandibular position.
Most authors agree that there is no single DVO with an exact value, but rather a comfort zone: DVO can therefore be modified within certain limits, thanks to muscular adaptation, although this is not fully understood in bruxers . [9,64]
The vertical dimension, which is related to neuromuscular balance, can vary according to physiological, psychological or pathological factors[5] . This is why the patient must be relaxed when determining the DV, as anxiety and fear cause the elevator muscles to contract[31] . In addition, the patient's position has an impact on the contraction of the masseter and temporalis muscles: it decreases when the patient is lying down, and increases sharply when the patient is seated, knees at 90° . [38]

3-6-2- Resting vertical dimension (DVR)

The vertical dimension of occlusion or postural equilibrium is characterized by the absence of inter-dental contact. It corresponds to the position occupied by the mandible when the patient's head is upright, the activity of the elevator and depressor muscles balances the forces of gravity, and the condyles are in a neutral position with no stress on the various anatomical components of the articular structures. Its value varies from one individual to another, and within the same individual over the course of a day.

3-6-3- Inocclusion space (ELI)

The free space is the distance between the occlusal surfaces of the maxillary and mandibular teeth when the mandible is in the resting position.

Numerous methods for determining this ELI are proposed in the literature: either direct methods (with measurement of the DVO) [77,86] or indirect methods (DVO measured from the DVR or ELI) . [36,53]

ELI plays an essential role in the neuromuscular balance of the stomatognathic system, guaranteeing proper orofacial function. Various studies show variations in this space (from 1 to 10 mm) [91] depending on age, skeletal type and posture, as well as physiological and psychological factors .[5]

Respecting this space is essential for the health of the occlusal system.

3-6-4- When to increase DVO?

The decision to increase DVO is based on physiological requirements for neuromuscular and/or prosthetic balance. Increasing the DVO allows us to re-establish this neuromuscular balance, to recreate a satisfactory inter-occlusal space to provide sufficient thickness for the prosthetic reconstruction (which will provide mechanical strength and improved esthetics), and to restore esthetics[5,7] . Increasing the DVO can only be done in cases of large prosthetic reconstructions[44] . When the DVO is reduced, it will be increased by rotating the mandible around the hinge axis[7] . There is therefore no reason to fear muscle dysfunctions if the occlusion is well managed[18] , even if the new DV exceeds the inocclusion clearance .[5]

The only precaution to be taken when increasing DVO is in patients with TMD: these should be normalized as a matter of priority, in order to achieve a reduction in signs and symptoms using reversible techniques. Similarly, in patients with marked osteoarthritis, a significant variation in DVO (more than 2mm at the incisal level) may cause joint stress .[64]

The increase in DVO rarely exceeds 3mm interincisally and therefore has little aesthetic or articular impact, but on the scale of the teeth this change is significant. Tooth visibility is assessed in the resting position: on average, 3mm visibility of maxillary teeth and 1mm of mandibular teeth meet aesthetic criteria .[44]

3-6-5- Preprosthetic proposal to create space

The pre-prosthetic clinical examination is essential for selecting the occlusal context in which the prosthetic restoration will be placed.

This step will determine the treatment plan and prognosis for future prosthetic work.

The initial occlusion will be preserved if there is no neuromuscular, articular or periodontal pathology, and if occlusal contacts are sufficiently well distributed and numerous.

The occlusion can be modified if there is no joint pathology or if the DVO is reduced.

Restructuring the occlusion corresponds to the creation of a position of maximum intercuspidity in centric relation.

In cases where the wear is significant but the DVO is unchanged with little free space, space must be created for the prosthetic restoration.

How do you create space?

❖ Use OIM-RC offset:

Moving from the position of maximum intercuspidia (MCI) to the position of centric relation (CR) can create anteriorly located space through mandibular proglation. The difference between ORC and OIM can be exploited when space is needed to treat severe wear on the palatal surfaces of the maxillary incisor-canine block and the vestibular surfaces of the mandibular incisors.

❖ Orthodontic treatment :

This treatment increases free space and aligns teeth. At the same time, it allows ingression, egression and translation movements.

❖ Coronary elongation:

A technique designed to lengthen the clinical crown in order to achieve a conservative or prosthetic dental restoration that respects the biological space. These objectives can only be achieved by taking into account the various biological, anatomical and aesthetic factors, which in turn determine the choice of appropriate technique (surgical or orthodontic). The aim is to preserve or re-establish a biological space compatible with good periodontal health, to enable better dentoprosthetic adaptation, to restore aesthetics and to guarantee the durability of the restoration . [37,55]

3-7- Occlusal reconstruction materials

The aim of occlusal reconstruction is to protect residual tooth structures and optimize occlusal function. The modifications made must be sparing to these dental structures while respecting an optimal benefit/risk ratio[34] . The practitioner will not treat superficial wear in the same way, rapid wear with loss of DVO, or slow, progressive wear with alveolar-dental erosion to compensate for the loss of DVO .[49]

In the case of bruxers, the choice of restorative biomaterial must meet aesthetic, biomechanical and conservative (minimally invasive) criteria, as well as compatibility with the bonding agent.

For these reasons, adhesive retention systems are recommended, with composite resins and ceramics (the material most likely to cause damage to occlusal structures when its finish or surface condition is inadequate) being the materials that best meet these criteria.

For reconstruction of posterior teeth: inlay/onlay, overlay (prosthetic part completely restoring the occlusal table), veneerlay (prosthetic part restoring the occlusal table and vestibular surface).

For the reconstruction of anterior teeth, we recommend the use of vestibular and/or palatal veneers (26,43) . For aesthetic reasons, vestibular veneers are generally made of ceramic(18) . They have the advantage of restoring both vestibular and free-edge wear, thus restoring the anterior guide in its entirety.

Practitioners today are talking about a new ENAMIC ceramic® : a unique hybrid ceramic with a dual ceramic-polymer network structure that appears to offer highly satisfactory characteristics and promising results, especially for the treatment of patients suffering from bruxism . (20,21)

Table III: Comparison of ceramic and resin properties.

<table>
<tr><th></th><th colspan="2">RESINE COMPOSITE</th><th>CERAMIQUE</th></tr>
<tr><td rowspan="3">+</td><td colspan="2">-Dureté proche de l'émail, minimise l'usure des dents antagonistes (70).
-Possibilité de réparation en cas de fracture (94),
-Résistance à la fatigue comparable à celle des céramiques (94)</td><td rowspan="3">-Esthétique +++
-Grande résistante mécanique (céramiques renforcées++).
-Possibilité de réalisation en technique CFAO
=> élimination de l'étape de laboratoire,
=> réalisation de restaurations en technique directe ou semi-directe au fauteuil.</td></tr>
<tr><td>Collage en méthode directe</td><td>Collage en méthode indirecte</td></tr>
<tr><td>-Moyen simple et de faible coût,
-Idéale pour restituer un léger sous-guidage.
-Succès de 90% après 30 mois, dans des cas de surélévation occlusale,
-Peut servir de test (évaluation, sans risques, de l'activité du bruxisme).</td><td>- Esthétique
-Meilleures propriétés mécaniques (résines composites hybrides +++)
-Meilleure biocompatibilité,
-Contraintes diminuées lors du retrait de polymérisation (CFAO +++).</td></tr>
<tr><td rowspan="2">−</td><td>-Rendu esthétique dans le temps.
-Difficulté de contrôle des morphologies sur le plan fonctionnel et sur le plan esthétique.</td><td colspan="2">-Demande des étapes de laboratoires,
-Coût plus élevé (cela même via la CFAO),
-Contrôle de collage précis (guide de collage).</td></tr>
<tr><td colspan="2">-Résistance limitée à l'usure des résines composites utilisées (renouvellement régulier du matériau à envisagé).</td><td>-Impossibilité de réparation en cas de fractures.</td></tr>
</table>

3-8- Transitional prosthesis

In the case of large-scale prosthetic reconstruction, it is necessary to test the patient's adaptability beforehand with a prosthesis close to the future prosthesis to be used. This provisional prosthesis is intended to be a faithful reproduction of the diagnostic wax.

In the case of a prosthetic treatment for a bruxing patient, its main role is to assess the feasibility of the future prosthetic project, as well as to observe any problems that may have arisen while wearing the prosthesis, so as to avoid failures when the final prosthesis is made. The prosthesis is made of baked resin and reinforced with metal to prevent it fracturing easily during an episode of bruxism.

According to Kois[42] , wearing the provisional prosthesis for 6 months allows us to test the neuro-musculo-articular adaptation capabilities of the manducatory apparatus, and also to confirm that the previously established vertical dimension of occlusion will not be iatrogenic.

According to some authors, the use of the provisional prosthesis during the production phase of the prosthesis in use is sufficient to validate the determined DVO, and it does not seem necessary to them to use it in the long term.

The temporary prosthesis can also be used to wait for gingival healing after surgery (coronal elongation). It helps to condition the tissues by preserving dento-periodontal relationships and avoiding inflammation - essential conditions for a quality impression.

It also enables the practitioner to monitor any loosening, fracture in which insufficient reduction of exaggerated muscle activity or a poorly chosen occlusal concept is suspected.

It is essential to monitor the patient during this temporary prosthetic phase. If ignored, they can compromise the durability of the final prosthesis.

In conclusion, the transitional prosthesis is an essential prerequisite that provides crucial information for the realization of definitive restorations, both in terms of the periodontal environment and from an esthetic and functional point of view. Only if the results after wear and control are satisfactory will the practitioner proceed with the realization of the definitive prosthesis .[32]

3-9- Prosthesis for use

Prosthetic fabrication[7] requires all the usual precautions[7] : cross-mounting (provisional and definitive bridges can be used equally as antagonists), use of silicone keys to reproduce provisional tooth shapes, programming of articulator condylar housings, individual incisal table and, of course, "a minima" guides and reduced cuspal slopes to avoid any occlusal problems.

Definitive prostheses can be made using either total or segmented reconstructions, where possible, to facilitate removal in the event of fissure or major fracture, or unitary reconstructions. Single-unit reconstructions are preferred for patients over 50 years of age, as the harmful masticatory forces are less significant. They also have the advantage of facilitating detection of prematurity, as the causal tooth will loosen rapidly .[85]

These patients require rigorous and regular follow-up. The protective occlusal splint must remain well-balanced, and the occlusal surfaces of reconstructions must be particularly closely observed, so as to be able to intervene if prosthetic occlusal morphologies change. Both the practitioner and the patient must never lose sight of the fact that prosthetic treatment does not act on the origins and causes of bruxism, but rather on its consequences.

3-10-Removable prosthesis

Removable prostheses can be used during treatment as transitional prostheses, enabling a new DVO to be tested while ensuring esthetics.

It can also be chosen when the prognosis of one or more teeth remains uncertain, thus allowing the progressive replacement of these teeth .[85]

Finally, it is indicated for patients with an unstable or pathological general condition .[65]

However, in certain cases of bruxism, this type of prosthesis is preferable to a fixed reconstruction. In such cases, overdenture restoration is possible. Abutments used in this way can be restored with a metal alloy inlay-core, or with an attachment to improve retention of the prosthesis.

These overdentures have their drawbacks. The roots remain susceptible to caries and periodontal disease, in which case the patient is advised to apply a fluoride gel under the denture and to visit the practice regularly for a check-up. The risk of root fracture is high during bruxism, when the roots are subjected to exaggerated pressure due to lateral forces.

Occlusal surfaces made of acrylic resin wear easily. Ceramic teeth can be considered, but in this case the wear of antagonistic teeth must be monitored. The removable and reversible nature of this type of prosthesis means it can be replaced at any time by a more aesthetic and comfortable fixed prosthesis.

3-11- Implant prosthesis and bruxism

In the absence of prospective, retrospective or epidemiological studies concerning a possible cause-and-effect relationship between bruxism, parafunctions and implant failure, it is not possible to conclude that there is a definite and absolute contraindication [51,96] . We must therefore anticipate potential problems as far as possible [15] , if we are not to be able to totally circumscribe their consequences. In practice, regular patient follow-up is essential.

The risk is that the supra-structure cannot deform beyond its elastic limit. In this case, occlusal forces may compromise osseointegration, leading to peri-implant resorption.[15]

According to Rangert[49] , around 75% of implant fractures occur in patients suffering from bruxism. He recommends the use of large-diameter implants in molar areas (>4mm).

Pre-implant analysis is used to choose between different prosthetic options. Available bone volume, occlusion, prosthetic needs and the patient's aesthetic requirements guide the prosthetic choice. Passive adaptation of the various components is essential. The insertion of the framework must be stress-free. From a biomechanical point of view, forces should ideally be distributed along the implant axis. Finally, the occlusal pattern selected must be designed to protect the implant with minimal guidance. . [81]

Conclusion

It would seem, then, that bruxism represents the exaggerated manifestation of a type of activity normally found in almost all individuals. Its detection and diagnosis are still based on empirical data, although it is relatively simple to establish in the sleep laboratory. Occlusal factors have long been considered the main cause of bruxism, but recent studies have shown a central origin.

Its multifactorial etiology makes it particularly difficult to treat, and it is currently impossible to completely prevent this para-functional activity. The practitioner faced with a bruxing patient must adopt a comprehensive, multidisciplinary and personalized approach.

According to Lobbezoo, the management of bruxism has three components according to the "**3P**" rule:

- **"Flat"**, corresponding to the use of occlusal splints.
- **"Pep Talk"**, which represents the behavioral approach.
- **"Pills"**, or pharmacological intervention, using centrally-acting drugs.

In cases where a prosthetic solution has become paramount, certain parameters need to be considered before any treatment begins, particularly the vertical dimension. These treatments will always be difficult, as the prosthetic restoration must not only meet aesthetic and functional requirements, but must also integrate with the parafunction.

Finally, regular monitoring is essential, especially in the case of major prosthetic work, to maintain the occlusal relationship chosen for the prosthesis in place.

References

1. **American Academy of Sleep Medicine.**
   International Classification of Sleep Disorders. 3rd ed.
   Westchester: American Academy of Sleep Medicine, 2014.
2. **Aoki R, Takaba M, Abe Y et al.**
   A pilot study to test the validity of a piezoelectric intra-splint force detector for monitoring of sleep bruxism in comparison to portable polysomnography.
   J Oral Sci 2022;64(1):63-8.
3. **Arzul L, Corre P, Khonsari RH, Mercier JM, Piot B.**
   Asymmetric hypertrophy of the masticatory muscles.
   Ann Chir Plast Esthet 2012;57(3):286-91.
4. **Bataillon T.**
   Bruxism: Strengthening cognitive-behavioral management through the development of a mobile application [Thesis].
   Marseille : Faculté d'Odontologie de Marseille, 2019.
5. **Blanchard JP, Bartala M.**
   Can we increase the vertical dimension of occlusion in fixed prosthesis?
   Paris: ADF, 1999:18-23.
6. **Bohnenkamp DM.**
   Removable partial dentures: clinical concepts.
   Dent Clin North Am 2014;58(1):69-89.
7. **Brocard D, Laluqe JF.**
   Bruxism and conjoint prosthesis: What attitudes to have?
   Cah Prothèse 1997;100:93-106.

8. **Brocard D, Lalluque JF, Knellsen C.**
Managing bruxism.
Paris: Quintessence International, 2007.

9. **Brocard D, Laluque JF, Knellesen C, Rozencweig DD.**
Managing bruxism.
Paris: Quintessence International, 2008.

10. **Chapotat B, Bailly F.**
Bruxism and prosthetic restorations.
Inf Dent 1999;38:2839-49.

11. **Chapotat B, Shenglin J, Robin O, Jouvet M.**
Sleep bruxism: fundamental and clinical aspects.
J Parodontol Implantol Orale 1999; 8:277-89.

12. **Charon J, Joachim F, Sandelé P.**
Parodontie clinique moderne.
Paris: CdP, 1994.

13. **Cherasia M, Parks L.**
Suggestions for use of behavioral measures in treating bruxism.
Psychol Rep 1986;58(3):719-22.

14. **Chikhani L, Dichamp J.**
Bruxism, algodysfunctional temporomandibular joint syndrome and botulinum toxin.
Ann Readapt Med Phys 2003;46(6):333-7.

15. **Chrcanovic BR, Kisch J, Albrektsson T, Wennerberg A.**
Bruxism and dental implant treatment complications: a retrospective comparative study of 98 bruxer patients and a matched group.
Clin Oral Implants Res 2017;28(7):1-9.

16. **D'InacauE.**

An anthropological approach to tooth wear.
Cah Prothèse 2004;126:19-32.

17. **D'Incau E, Micoulaud-Franchi JA, Brocard D, Laluque JF.**
Validity of the diagnosis of sleep bruxism.
Rev Odontstomatol 2017;46:222-39.

18. **Dahl BL, Carlsson GE, Ekfeldt A.**
Occlusal wear of teeth and restorative materials.
Acta Odontol Scand 1993;(51):299-311.

19. **De Boever JA, Carlsson GE, Klineberg IJ.**
Need for occlusal therapy and prosthodontic treatment in the management of temporomandibular disorders. Part I. Occlusal interferences and occlusal adjustment.
J Oral Rehabil 2000;27(5):367-79.

20. **Dirxen C, Blunck U, Preissner S.**
Clinical performance of a new biomimetic double network material.
Open Dent J 2013;7:118-22.

21. **Djemal S, Darbar UR, Hemmings KW.**
Case report: tooth wear associated with an unusual habit.
Eur J Prosthodont Restor Dent 1998;6(1):29-32.

22. **Duminil G.**
Extensive occlusal rehabilitation: principles. In: Duminil G, Orthlieb JD, Bolla M et al, eds. Le Bruxisme tout simplement.
Paris: Espace ID, 2015:271-88.

23. **Dylina TJ.**
A common-sense approach to splint therapy.
J Prosthet Dent 2001;86(5):539-45.

24. **Ekberg E, Vallon D, Nilner M.**
The efficacy of appliance therapy in patients with temporomandibular

disorders of mainly myogenous origin. A randomized, controlled, short-term trial.
J Orofac Pain 2003;17(2):133-9.

25. **Ella B, Ghorayeb I, Burbaud P, Guehl D.**
Bruxism in movement disorders: A comprehensive review.
J Prosthodont 2017;26(7):599-605.

26. **Etienne O, Toledano C.**
Minimally invasive rehabilitations. In: Duminil G, Orthlieb JD et al. Le Bruxisme tout simplement.
Paris: Espace ID, 2015:253-70.

27. **Farquhar M, Urquhart DS, Russo K et al.**
Response to 'How to interpret polysomnography' by Leong et al.
Arch Dis Child Educ Pract Ed 2020;105(3):136.

28. **Fleiter B, Estrade D.**
Reference position and disc dysfunction. In: Positions de référence? Choix, acquisition, maintien.
Paris, CNO, 1997:41-50.

29. **Frank DL, Khorshid L, Kiffer JF, Moravec CS, McKee MG.**
Biofeedback in medicine: who, when, why and how?
Ment Health Fam Med 2010;7(2):85-91.

30. **Freund B, Schwartz M, Symington JM.**
Botulinum toxin: new treatment for temporomandibular disorders.
Br J Oral Maxillofac Surg 2000;38(5):466-71.

31. **Garrido-Delorme M.**
Prosthetic considerations in the bruxism patient [Thesis].
Bordeaux: UFR des Sciences Odontologiques de Bordeaux, 2014.

32. **Geoffrion J.**
Single- and multiple-unit fixed prosthesis: difficult cases and their

clinical solutions.
Chir Dent Fr 1998;907:32-4.

33. **Giggins OM, Persson UM, Caulfield B.**
Biofeedback in rehabilitation.
J Neuroeng Rehabil 2013;10:60.

34. **Giraudeau A, Ehrmann E, Orthlieb JD, LaplancheO.**
Example of preprosthetic management of a "bruxer" patient.
Inf Dent 2014:12-9.

35. **Gremillion HA, Klasser GD.**
Temporomandibular disorders: Priorities for research and care.
Washington : National Academies Press, 2020.

36. **Gross MD, Ormianer Z.**
A preliminary study on the effect of occlusal vertical dimension increase on mandibular postural rest position.
Int J Prosthodont 1994;7(3):216-26.

37. **Hayon L.**
Restoration of biological space by surgical coronal elongation or orthodontic egression: indications and therapeutic choices.
J Parodontol Implant Orale 2005;24(3):187-96.

38. **Helfer M, Demengel P, Vermande G.**
Restoration of function and esthetics using combined prostheses.
Prosthetic Strategy 2013;13(2):1-10.

39. **Jafari B, Mohsenin V.**
Polysomnography.
Clin Chest Med 2010;31(2):287-97.

40. **Jung Ho Kim, Padraig McAuliffe, BrianO'Connel, Dermot**

Diamond.

Development of Bite Guard for Wireless Monitoring of Bruxism Using Pressure-Sensitive Polymer.

Conference: International Conference on Body Sensor Networks, BSN 2010, Singapore, 7-9 June, 2010.

41. **Kaleka R, Saporta S, Bouter D, Bonte E.**

Cervical wear lesions (CWL): Etiopathogenesis.

Real Clin 2001;12(4):367-85.

42. **Kim JJ.**

Revisiting the removable partial denture.

Dent Clin North Am 2019;63(2):263-78.

43. **Kois JC.**

Restoring or modifying the vertical dimension of occlusion: controversies.

12 èmes Journées internationales du CNO.

Paris: CNO, 1995:185-98.

44. **Lambrechts P, Van Meerbeek B, Perdigão J, Gladys S, Braem M, Vanherle G.**

Restorative therapy for erosive lesions.

Eur J Oral Sci 1996;104(2):229-40.

45. **Laurent M, Touchet T.**

Vertical dimension variation and prosthetic therapy: clinical illustrations.

Real Clin 2013;24(2):139-45.

46. **Lauret JF, Le Gall MG.**

La mastication, une réalité par l'occluso-odontologie?

The occlusal function mastication 1997;85:31-50.

47. **Lavigne GJ, Goulet JP, Zuconni M, Morrison F, Lobbezoo F.**

Sleep disorders and the dental patient: an overview.
Oral Surg Oral Med Oral Pathol Oral Radiol Endod 1999;88(3):257-72.

48. **Lobbezoo F, Ahlberg J, Glaros AG et al.**
Bruxism defined and graded: an international consensus.
J Oral Rehabil 2013;40(1):2-4.

49. **Lobbezoo F, Lavigne GJ.**
Do bruxism and temporomandibular disorders have a cause-and-effect relationship?
J Orofac Pain 1997;11(1):15-23.

50. **Lobbezoo F, van der Zaag J, van Selms MK, Hamburger HL, Naeije M.**
Principles for the management of bruxism.
J Oral Rehabil 2008;35(7):509-23.

51. **Long H, Liao Z, Wang Y, Liao L, Lai W.**
Efficacy of botulinum toxins on bruxism: an evidence-based review.
Int Dent J 2012;62(1):1-5.

52. **Manfredini D, Poggio CE, Lobbezoo F.**
Is bruxism a risk factor for dental implants? A systematic review of the literature.
Clin Implant Dent Relat Res 2014;16(3):460-9.

53. **Manfredini D, Serra-Negra J, Carboncini F, Lobbezoo F.**
Current concepts of bruxism.
Int J Prosthodont 2017;30(5):437-8.

54. **Meier B, Luck O, Harzer W.**
Interocclusal clearance during speech and in mandibular rest position. A comparison between different measuring methods.
J Orofac Orthop 2003;64(2):121-34.

55. **Monaco A, Sgolastra F, Pietropaoli D, Giannoni M, Cattaneo R.**
Comparison between sensory and motor transcutaneous electrical nervous stimulation on electromyographic and kinesiographic activity of patients with temporomandibular disorder: a controlled clinical trial.
BMC Musculoskelet Disord 2013;14:168.

56. **Monnet-Corti V, Glise JM.**
Surgical coronary elongation.
Clinic 2004;25(4):209-12.

57. **Muñoz Lora VRM, Del Bel Cury AA, Jabbari B, Lacković Z.**
Botulinum toxin type A in dental medicine.
J Dent Res 2019;98(13):1450-7.

58. **Nishigawa K, Kondo K, Takeuchi H, Clark GT.**
Contingent electrical lip stimulation for sleep bruxism: a pilot study.
J Prosthet Dent 2003;89(4):412-7.

59. **Ocransky SS.**
The bacterial etiology of destructive periodontal disease: Current concepts.
J Periodontal 1992;63:322-31.

60. **Oliveira SSI, Pannuti CM, Paranhos KS et al.**
Effect of occlusal splint and therapeutic exercises on postural balance of patients with signs and symptoms of temporomandibular disorder.
Clin Exp Dent Res 2019;5(2):109-15.

61. **Omar R.**
Reappraising prosthodontic treatment goals for older, partially dentate people: Part I. Traditional management strategy.
SADJ 2004;59(5):198-202.

62. **Omar R.**

Reappraising prosthodontic treatment goals for older, partially dentate people: Part II. Case for a sustainable dentition?
SADJ 2004;59(6):228-34.

63. **Onodera K, Kawagoe T, Sasaguri K, Protacio-Quismundo C, Sato S.**
The use of a bruxchecker in the evaluation of different grinding patterns during sleep bruxism.
Cranio 2006;24(4):292-9.

64. **Orthlieb JD, Cheynet F.**
Orthèses (Gouttières) occlusales : indications dans les Dysfonctions Temporo-Mandibulaires - Recommandations de Bonne Pratique.
Conference: Société Française de Stomatologie, Chirurgie Maxillo-Faciale et Chirurgie, January 2016.

65. **Orthlieb JD, Rebibo M, Mantout B.**
The vertical dimension of occlusion in fixed prosthetics. Critères de décision.
Cah Prothèse 2002;120:67-80.

66. **Packer ME, Davis DM.**
The long-term management of patients with tooth surface loss treated using removable appliances.
Dent Update 2000;27(9):454-8.

67. **Paesani DA.**
Bruxism: Theory and practice.
New Malden: Quintessence Publishing, 2010.

68. **Quemar JC, Rozenczweig D.**
Reference position? Choix, acquisition, maintien.
Compte rendu des 14èmes journées internationales du collège

national d'occlusodontologie.
Paris, CNO, 1997:95.

69. **Quintero Y, Restrepo CC, Tamayo V et al.**
Effect of awareness through movement on the head posture of bruxist children.
J Oral Rehabil 2009;36(1):18-25.

70. **Ré JP.**
Les gouttière occlusale. In: Duminil G, Orthlieb JD, Bolla M et al, eds. Le Bruxisme tout simplement.
Paris: Espace ID, 2015:215-26.

71. **Ré JP.**
Orthèses orales Gouttières occlusales, Apnées du sommeil et ronflements, Protège-dents. Guide Clinique.
Paris: CdP, 2011.

72. **Ré JP, Chossegros C, El Zoghby A, Carlier JF, Orthlieb JD.**
Gouttières occlusales. Mise au point.
Rev Stomatol Chir Maxillofac 2009;110(3):145-9.

73. **Rodrigues D, Siriani AO, Bérzin F.**
Effect of conventional TENS on pain and electromyographic activity of masticatory muscles in TMD patients.
Braz Oral Res 2004;18(4):290-5.

74. **Rozencweig D.**
Algies et dysfonctionnement de l'appareil manducateur.
Paris: CdP, 1994.

75. **Rozencweig D.**

Bruxism, an ongoing challenge to our treatments.
Inf Dent 2002;84:2893-8.

76. Rugh JD, Harlan J.
Nocturnal bruxism and temporomandibular disorders.
Adv Neurol 1988;49:329-41.

77. Saczuk K, Lapinska B, Wilmont P, Pawlak L, Lukomska-Szymanska M.
The bruxoff device as a screening method for sleep bruxism in dental practice.
J Clin Med 2019;8(7):930.

78. Samoian R.
The vertical dimension of the lower face.
Grenoble: R. Samoian, 1984.

79. Sarfati E, Radiguet J.
Occlusal diagrams in fixed prosthetics.
Actual Odonto-Stomatol 2007;100:247-60.

80. Sato M, Iizuka T, Watanabe A, Iwase N, Otsuka H, Terada N, Fujisawa M.
Electromyogram biofeedback training for daytime clenching and its effect on sleep bruxism.
J Oral Rehabil 2015;42(2):83-9.

81. Sato S, Hotta TH, Pedrazzi V.
Removable occlusal overlay splint in the management of tooth wear: a clinical report.
J Prosthet Dent 2000;83(4):392-5.

82. Simonet P, Duminil G.
Bruxism and implantology. In: Duminil G, Orthlieb JD, Bolla M et al,

eds. Le Bruxisme tout simplement.
Paris: Espace ID, 2015:303-16.

83. **Sugimoto K, Yoshimi H, Sasaguri K, Sato S.**
Occlusion factors influencing the magnitude of sleep bruxism activity.
Cranio 2011;29(2):127-37.

84. **Tago C, Aoki S, Sato S.**
Status of occlusal contact during sleep bruxism in patients who visited dental clinics - A study using a Bruxchecker®.
Cranio 2018;36(3):167-73.

85. **Tinastepe N, Küçük BB, Oral K.**
Botulinum toxin for the treatment of bruxism.
Cranio 2015;33(4):291-8.

86. **Treacy K.**
Awareness/relaxation training and transcutaneous electrical neural stimulation in the treatment of bruxism.
J Oral Rehabil 1999;26(4):280-7.

87. **Tryde G, McMillan DR, Christensen J, Brill N.**
The fallacy of facial measurements of occlusal height in edentulous subjects.
J Oral Rehabilitation 1976;3(4):353-8.

88. **Unger F.**
Management of temporomandibular disorders. The role of occlusal splints.
Rev Stomatol Chir Maxillofac 2001;102(1):47-54.

89. **Vavrina J, Vavrina J.**
Bruxism: Classification, Diagnostics and Treatment.

Praxis 2020;109(12):973-8.

90. von Gonten AS, Rugh JD.
Nocturnal muscle activity in the edentulous patient with and without dentures.
J Prosthet Dent 1984;51(5):709-13.

91. Watson TS.
Effectiveness of arousal and arousal plus overcorrection to reduce nocturnal bruxism.
J Behav Ther Exp Psychiatry 1993;24(2):181-5.

92. Watt DM, MacGregor AR.
Designing complete dentures.
Philadelphia: Saunders, 1976.

93. Wichniak A, Wierzbicka A, Walęcka M, Jernajczyk W.
Effects of antidepressants on sleep.
Curr Psychiatry Rep 2017;19(9):63.

94. Winocur E, Gavish A, Voikovitch M, Emodi-Perlman A, Eli I.
Drugs and bruxism: a critical review.
J Orofac Pain 2003;17(2):99-111.

95. Woda A, Pionchon P.
Mandibular postures and reference positions. Compte rendu du CNO.
Paris: CNO, 1997:19-40.

96. Yip KH, Chow TW, Chu FC.
Rehabilitating a patient with bruxism-associated tooth tissue loss: a literature review and case report.
Gen Dent 2003;51(1):70-6.

97. Zhou Y, Gao J, Luo L, Wang Y.

Does bruxism contribute to dental implant failure? a systematic review and meta-analysis.

Clin Implant Dent Relat Res 2016;18(2):410-20.

Internet references

98. Dental Visionist.

Hybrid ceramics in practice: A CAD/CAM material for patients with functional disorders? [Online].

[Accessed 15/02/2021], available from URL: https://www1.dental-visionist.com/en/A-CADCAM-material-for-patients-with-functional-disorders-263.html?kategorie=622

99. Kinessonne.com.

Le biofeedback [Online].

[Accessed 18/01/2021], available from URL: https://www.kinessonne.com/blog-kinessonne/index.php?post/2016/10/26/Le-biofeedback

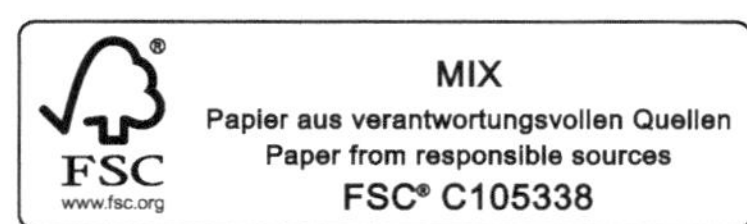

Printed by Books on Demand GmbH, Norderstedt / Germany